Needs and prospects of child and
adolescent psychiatry

Needs and Prospects of Child and Adolescent Psychiatry

Needs and Prospects of
Child and Adolescent Psychiatry

Edited by

MARTIN H. SCHMIDT
University of Heidelberg
Central Institute of Mental Health, Mannheim

and

HELMUT REMSCHMIDT
University of Marburg

Hogrefe & Huber Publishers
Toronto • Lewiston, NY • Bern • Göttingen • Stuttgart

R J
499
.N34
1989

Library of Congress Cataloging-in-Publication Data

Needs and prospects of child and adolescent psychiatry / Martin H. Schmidt,
Helmut Remschmidt (editors).
    p. cm.
    Proceedings of a symposium.
    Includes bibliographies

1. Child psychiatry—Congresses. 2. Adolescent psychiatry—Congresses.
I. Schmidt, Martin H. II. Remschmidt, Helmut.
[DNLM: 1. Adolescent Psychiatry—congresses. 2. Child Psychiatry—congresses.
3. Mental Disorders—in adolescence—congresses. 4. Mental Disorders—in
infancy & childhood—congresses. WS 350 N375]
RJ499.N34   1989   618.92'89—dc19

Canadian Cataloguing in Publication Data

Main entry under title:

Needs and prospects of child and adolescent psychiatry

Bibliography: p.

1. Child psychiatry. 2. Adolescent psychiatry. 3. Child psychiatry—Research.
4. Adolescent psychiatry—Research. I. Schmidt, Martin H. II. Remschmidt,
Helmut.

RJ499.N43   1989   618.92'89   C89-093395-2

© Copyright 1989 by Hans Huber Publishers

P. O. Box 51
Lewiston, NY   14092

12–14 Bruce Park Ave.
Toronto, Ontario M4P 2S3

Printed in Germany

ISBN 0-920887-55-4
Hans Huber Publishers • Toronto • Lewiston, NY • Bern • Stuttgart
ISBN 3-456-81808-4
Hans Huber Publishers • Bern • Stuttgart • Toronto • Lewiston, NY

Editors' Preface

Current medical care would be unthinkable without child and adolescent psychiatry as a discipline of its own. As in other branches, measures taken in child and adolescent psychiatry are derived from experiences that, ideally, should be subjected to empirical testing. This demand to scrutinize the experiences underlying medical treatment, however, is only partly accomplished. This applies not only to child and adolescent psychiatry, although—as a rather young discipline—it does have a multifarious empirical deficit. Yet new research findings and improved laboratory data are continuously enlarging our knowledge and giving us new guidelines for practical action—even if they at the same time unearth research deficits. A field like child and adolescent psychiatry is prone to adhere to ideologies, and this again undermines the necessity to refer to solid facts buttressed by empirical studies.

Not all findings of empirical studies can be easily and quickly translated into action, that is, medical practice. This may be more easily possible in the field of diagnostics, but it is rather difficult in the field of therapy, and even more so in the field of prevention. And these problems of gaining and transferring knowledge arise all the more in developing countries with insufficient child psychiatric facilities and tradition. Thus, defining relevant research topics not only requires looking out for "uncultivated terrain," it also means concentrating on the most important topics.

A meeting in March 1988 of about 40 scientists from Europe and the United States, supported by the West German Federal Ministry of Research and Technology and by the World Health Organization (WHO), was devoted to this problem of defining the priorities of future research. The recommendations were directed toward both the improvement of child psychiatric research in Germany and a general transfer to as many other countries as possible in order to achieve the greatest possible benefit for children and adolescents suffering from very common and/or severe and long-lasting psychiatric disorders. The meeting was mainly directed toward the topics of multilevel research, research on maturational problems, therapy evaluation, and prevention research, which seemed to be of utmost importance. The main purpose of this enterprise was to review the state of relevant subfields of child and adolescent psychiatric research with the intent of deriving those questions most urgently calling for an answer, and to point to viable ways and promising strategies of finding an answer to these problems. This is how the presented volume originated. The papers were conceived to pave the way for recommendations on future steps that should be taken in order to advance our knowledge.

From this view—in our opinion—priority should be given to

1) multilevel research on the stability and on change in child and adolescent psychiatric disorders,

2) research on externalizing disorders,

3) research on developmental disorders, and

4) intervention research concerning both special forms of treatment and prevention and the health system as a whole.

It is thus our recommendation to the Ministry of Research and Technology that special funding be provided for research projects studying these topics. It is our hope that these recommendations will provide a fresh impetus to research in child and adolescent psychiatry and will encourage fruitful research activities.

We wish to thank the authors for having devoted their contributions to this effort. Their scientific reputation guarantees that the goal in mind can indeed be achieved. Our special thanks go to the Minister of Research and Technology for his financial support, to the World Health Organization for its co-sponsorship, to Hans Huber Publishers (in particular to J.A. Smith) for its support in the publication of this volume as well as to Ms. Petra Möcks for her assistance in the editorial work.

The editors sincerely hope the present volume will aid in the translation of the recommendations in actual scientific research, and thus also help to develop child and adolescent psychiatry in clinical practice as well as in empirical research.

Martin H. Schmidt   March 1989
Helmut Remschmidt

Foreword

In most countries of the world, children account for some 50% of the population. It is, therefore, of utmost importance that their psychiatric needs be given the priority they deserve. It is unfortunate that because children are anyway in a position of being dependent on adults, the increased dependency that accompanies psychiatric disability is accepted with little questioning, few resources being made available to help the children and their families. It is still a fact that it is *adults* with psychiatric needs who command most of the resources available in mental health services. A symposium such as the one presented in this volume is thus important in highlighting the psychiatric needs of children.

The World Health Organization (WHO) is carrying out several activities related to child mental health and psychosocial development as well as child psychiatry within its Mental Health Program. The report of a WHO Expert Committee on this subject published in 1977 is still very pertinent and worthy of study[1]. The WHO is also working on a number of projects aimed at promoting the psychological well-being of children and adolescents as well as preventing psychological disorders. In this respect, a survey is being made of intervention techniques that can be used in promoting psychosocial skills among this group. In particular, it would be expected that this would lead to less antisocial behavior, less self-damaging, risk-taking behavior, and less later psychopathology. While it is easier to introduce such interventions in schools, the WHO is mindful of the fact that in many countries of the world a large number of children get little or no schooling, and that children who are not attending school are, in any case, those at highest risk.

Legislation can also be an instrument in promoting good mental health and in preventing psychosocial harm. The WHO, therefore, works together with governments around the globe to examine and amend legislation, especially where it affects children, in order to ensure optimal benefits for the well-being of such children.

In recent years, the WHO has produced some prototype manuals on child mental health for various levels of health workers in developing countries[2]. The WHO has also developed and pilot-tested a set of criteria for quality control of child day-care centers[3].

More specifically in the field of child psychiatry, the proposed ICD 10 will reflect the most up-to-date thinking concerning diagnosis, and a revised psychosocial axis for a multiaxial classification of child psychiatric disorders has been prepared for pilot testing[4].

As for services for children and adolescents, the WHO is encouraging the introduction of relevant aspects of child psychiatry into primary health care programs. It has to be realized, however, that for the developing countries of the world the long, elaborate, and detailed assessments and interventions found in the developed world are inappropriate. The funds available to deal with the problems amount to only a few dollars per case, and the time available is in the order of minutes rather than hours. It is therefore important for those giving advice on this subject to examine their own knowledge and skills and determine what can indeed be given to those with less education to use during a short consultation. For the world as a whole, therefore, an important area of research in the developed world is to identify these components of service that can be applied in the developing countries, bearing in mind the differences in culture and the scarcity of skilled professional resources. Nevertheless, the wealth of other human resources in such countries can make up for this deficiency, especially with the provision of some simple technologies which can be used in those situations.

Dr. J. Orley, Senior Medical Officer, Division of Mental Health, World Health Organization

---

[1] WHO Expert Committee on Child Mental Health and Psychosocial Development. Seventeenth Report. (1977). Geneva: World Health Organization. 71 pages. (World Health Organization Technical Report Series, No. 613).

[2] Manual on child mental health and psychosocial development. Part I: For the primary health care physician (5 March 1982). SEA/Ment/65.
Manual on child mental health and psychosocial development. Part II: For the primary health worker (20 April 1982). SEA/Ment/66. Restricted.
Manual on child mental health and psychosocial development. Part III: For teachers. (1982). SEA/Ment/67.
Manual on child mental health and psychosocial development. Part IV: For workers in children's homes. (1982) SEA/Ment/68..

[3] User's Manual for Child Care Facility Schedule—Draft for pilot testing. MNH/PRO/86.2 (A) (E, F).
Child Care Facility Schedule—Draft for pilot testing. MNH/PRO/86.2 (B) (E, F).

[4] World Health Organization. (1988). Multiaxial Classification of Child Psychiatric Disorders. Axis Five. Associated Abnormal Psychosocial Situations. Geneva: World Health Organization. 45 pages. (MNH/PRO/86.1. Rev. 1).

Table of Contents

SECTION III:
PERSPECTIVES OF INTERVENTION RESEARCH

Part 1: Epidemiological Basis

Part 2: Evaluation Research

Part 3: Long-Term Effects of Intervention

SECTION IV:
PERSPECTIVES OF PREVENTION RESEARCH

Part 1: Prediction—Starting Point of Prevention

Part 2: Evaluation Research in the Field of Prevention

Part 3: Putting Preventive Knowledge into Practice

List of Contributors

T. M. Achenbach
The University of Vermont
College of Medicine
Department of Psychiatry
1 South Prospect Street
Burlington, Vermont 05401
USA

F. Almqvist
Leavägen 7 B
SF–02700 Grankulla
Finland

J. C. Anthony
The Johns Hopkins University
School of Hygiene and Public
Health
Department of Mental Hygiene
615 North Wolfe Street
Baltimore, Maryland 21205
USA

V. Bell
Newcastle Health Authority
The Fleming Nuffield Unit
(For Children and Young People)
Burdon Terrace
GB–Newcastle upon Tyne NE2
3AX
England

M. Bohman
Umea Universitet
Barn- och ungdomspsychiatriska
kliniken
S–901 85 Umea
Sweden

C. H. Brown
The Johns Hopkins University
School of Hygiene and Public
Health
Department of Mental Hygiene
615 North Wolfe Street
Baltimore, Maryland 21205
USA

C. R. Cloninger
Umea Universitet
Barn- och ungdomspsychiatriska
kliniken
S–901 85 Umea
Sweden

A. D. Cox
Department of Psychiatry
Child and Adolescent Psychiatry
and Psychology
Royal Liverpool Children's Hospital
Alder Hey
Eaton Road
GB–Liverpool L12 2AP
England

L. Dolan
The Johns Hopkins University
School of Hygiene and Public
Health
Department of Mental Hygiene
615 North Wolfe Street
Baltimore, Maryland 21205
USA

H. van Engeland
Department of Child and
Adolescent Psychiatry
University of Utrecht
Nicolaas Beetstraat 24
NL–3511 GV Utrecht
The Netherlands

C. Gillberg
Göteborgs Universitet
Barnneuropsykiatriskt Centrum
Box 17113
S–402 61 Göteborg
Sweden

P. J. Graham
Department of Child Psychiatry
Institute of Child Health
The Hospital for Sick Children
Great Ormond Street
GB–London WC1N 3JH
England

R. E. Ingram
Doctoral Training Facility
Psychology Annex for Research
and Training
San Diego State University
6363 Alvarado Court, Suite 103
San Diego, CA 92182-0551
USA

S. G. Kellam
The Johns Hopkins University
School of Hygiene and Public
Health
Department of Mental Hygiene
615 North Wolfe Street
Baltimore, Maryland 21205
U.S.A

C. Klicpera
Institut für Psychologie
Abteilung für Angewandte Psychologie
Gölsdorfg. 3/6
A–1010 Wien
Austria

I. Kolvin
Newcastle Health Authority
The Fleming Nuffield Unit
(For Children and Young People)
Burdon Terrace
GB–Newcastle upon Tyne NE2
3AX
England

S. Lyne
Newcastle Health Authority
The Fleming Nuffield Unit
(For Children and Young People)
Burdon Terrace
GB–Newcastle upon Tyne NE2
3AX
England

A. Macmillam
University of Leicester
Department of Child Psychiatry
Clinical Science Building
Leicester Royal Infirmary,PO Box
65
GB–Leicester LE2 7LX
England

J. Martinius
Institut für Kinder- u.
Jugendpsychiatrie
der Ludwig-Maximilians-Universität
Heckscher Klinik
Heckscherstr. 4
D–8000 München 40
Federal Republic of Germany

A. R. Nicol
University of Leicester
Department of Child Psychiatry

Clinical Science Building
Leicester Royal Infirmary,PO Box
65
GB–Leicester LE2 7LX
England

J. Orley
Senior Medical Officer
Devision of Mental Health
World Health Organisation
CH–1211 Geneva 27
Switzerland

F. Poustka
Abt. für Kinder- und Jugendpsychiatrie an der
Johann Wolfgang Goethe-Universität
Deutschordenstraße 50
D–6000 Frankfurt/Main 70
Federal Republic of Germany

H. Remschmidt
Klinik und Poliklinik für
Kinder- und Jugendpsychiatrie
der
Philipps-Universität Marburg
Hans-Sachs-Str. 6
D-3550 Marburg
Federal Republic of Germany

L. N. Robins
Department of Psychiatry
Washington University School of
Medicine
Medical School Box 8134
4940 Audubon Avenue
St. Louis, Missouri 63110
USA

J. E. Rolf
The Johns Hopkins University
School of Hygiene and Public
Health
615 North Wolfe Road
Baltimore, Maryland 21205
USA

A. Rothenberger
Kinder- und Jugendpsychiatrische Klinik
Zentralinstitut für Seelische Gesundheit
J5
D–6800 Mannheim 1
Federal Republic of Germany

M. H. Schmidt
Kinder- und Jugendpsychi-
atrische Klinik
Zentralinstitut für Seelische Ge-
sundheit
J5
D-6800 Mannheim 1
Federal Republic of Germany

S. Sigvardsson
Umea Universitet
Barn- och ungdomspsychiatriska
kliniken
S–901 85 Umea
Sweden

R. K. Silbereisen
Justus-Liebig-Universität Gießen
Fachbereich 06 Psychologie
Otto-Behaghel Str. 10
D-6300 Gießen
Federal Republic of Germany

I. Spurkland
Child Psychiatric Clinic
University of Oslo
Box 59, Vinderen
Oslo 3
Norway

E. Taylor
Department of Child and Adoles-
cent Psychiatry
Institute of Psychiatry
De Crespigny Park, Denmark Hill
GB–London SE5 8AF
England

Y. Tsiantis
Department of Psychological Pae-
diatrics
Aghia Sophia Children's Hospital
Athens 115 27
Greece

F. C. Verhulst
Kinder- en jeugdpsychiatrie

sophia kinderziekenhuis
gordelweg 160
NL–3038 GE Rotterdam
The Netherlands

A. Warnke
Klinik und Poliklinik für
Kinder- und Jugendpsychiatrie
der Philipps-Universität
Hans-Sachs-Str. 6
D–3550 Marburg
Federal Republic of Germany

L. Werthamer-Larsson
The Johns Hopkins University
School of Hygiene and Public
Health
Department of Mental Hygiene
615 North Wolfe Street
Baltimore, Maryland 21205
USA

R. Wilson
The Johns Hopkins University
School of Hygiene and Public
Health
Department of Mental Hygiene
615 North Wolfe Street
Baltimore, Maryland 21205
USA

S. N. Wolkind
The Maudsley Hospital
Denmark Hill
GB–London SE5 8AZ
England

F. Wolstenholme
University of Leicester
Department of Child Psychiatry
Clinical Science Building
Leicester Royal Infirmary
PO Box 65
GB–Leicester LE2 7LX
England

SECTION I:

CONCEPTUAL AND METHODOLOGICAL APPROACHES

Developmental Psychopathology as a Theoretical Framework for Child and Adolescent Psychiatry

Helmut Remschmidt*

Developmental Psychopathology as an Integrative Discipline

There can be no doubt that the developmental perspective is of great importance for the understanding of psychiatric disturbances in children and adolescents. Developmental physiology, developmental neurology, and developmental psychology are basic sciences of child psychiatry. The developmental perspective can be looked upon as a kind of bridge between the different disciplines or as a unifying concept (Eisenberg, 1977), integrating different scientific and practical approaches to normality and psychopathology, not only for children, but also for adults. Though there is general agreement about this view, we are far away from a comprehensive and substantial theory of development that would be able to integrate earlier and recent knowledge—and at the same time be open to new hypotheses and results.

Yet, the developmental perspective is not a new one. Looking through the history of child psychiatry and psychopathology, I found the first hint on the developmental aspect in the German textbook by Hermann Emminghaus (1887) with the title *Psychic Disturbances of Childhood*. There, Emminghaus writes, after complaining that there is no systematic and general symptomatology of childhood psychoses, that it is the task of psychopathology to study the anomalies of the mind through all developmental stages and to differentiate normal from pathological psychic processes (Emminghaus, 1887, p. 4).

Also, the famous textbook written by August Homburger (1926) starts with a chapter on "Normal and deviant development in childhood," using categories such as "retarded and delayed development," "accelerated and premature development," "disturbed and broken development," and "deviant de-

* *Acknowledgement:* I would like to thank Dr. C. Gutenbrunner, Dipl.-Math. for his assistance in the construction of models.

velopment by deviant disposition." As well the textbooks by Leo Kanner (1935) and Moritz Tramer (1941) include the developmental perspective, followed by the books of J. Feldner (1955) with the title *Developmental Psychiatry of Childhood*; Tom Achenbach (1974; 2nd ed. 1982) *Developmental Psychopathology*; and Michael Rutter (1980) *Developmental Psychiatry*. Meanwhile, there also exist several other volumes on the topic.

Nevertheless, the emergence of developmental psychopathology was characterized by "adultomorphism," which means a tendency to understand psychiatric disorders of childhood as predecessors of analogously named disturbances in adults.

According to Sroufe and Rutter (1984, p. 18), the basic perspectives of developmental psychopathology are as follows:

1. The discipline "is concerned with development and is therefore closely wedded to the whole of developmental psychology." Logically, developmental psychopathology thus has to use the methods, theories, and perspectives of developmental psychology.

2. The second topic is the focus on psychopathology, which means looking primarily at developmental deviations.

3. The third element is, in my view, the integrative perspective, including and combining biological, psychological, and psychosocial approaches with respect to all structures and functions in the growing child.

Table 1. Potential relationship between psychopathology and developmental tasks (Garber, 1984).

Psychopathological Disorder	Developmental Task
Separation anxiety	Object permanence, attachment and dependency
Depression	Differentiation of self, self-esteem, social comparison
Suicide	Concept of death, time perspective (future)
Conduct disorder:	
Undersocialized	Moral development
Aggressive	Perspective-taking, empathy
Impulsivity	Delay of gratification
Oppositional disorder	Autonomy, individuation
Schizoid disorder	Peer relations, friendship patterns

Taking these elements into consideration, we may define developmental psychopathology as "the study of the origins and course of individual patterns of behavioral maladaptation whatever the age of onset, whatever the causes, whatever the transformations in behavioral manifestation, and however complex the course of the developmental pattern may be" (Sroufe & Rutter, 1984, p. 18).

Another definition, given by Rolf and Read (1984, p. 9) runs as follows: "The term 'developmental psychopathology' can be defined as the study of abnormal behavior within a context of measuring the effects of genetic, ontogenetic, biochemical, cognitive, affective, social or any other ongoing developmental influences on behavior."

Both definitions stress the integrative aspect, and from this point of view, developmental psychopathology "is the product of an integration of various disciplines the efforts of which had previously been separated and distinct" (Cicchetti, 1984, p. 1).

In this sense, developmental psychopathology can be characterized by the following principles:

1. We can learn more about psychopathology if we better understand normal development. In this view, psychopathology can be understood as a distortion or exaggeration of normal development.

2. We can learn more about normal functioning of an organism by studying psychopathology.

3. To understand all these aspects in children, we have to study their behavior under the perspective of development.

Bearing these principles in mind, we can say that the developmental perspective includes processes such as growth, maturation, learning as well as the interactions between and among these influences. But one has also to realize that not all influences on children have to do with development; accidental influences exist as well, impairments and unfavorable conditions that are as such not developmental factors, though they do influence development in a profound way. The changes in development are age-related and consist of transformations in the structure and the function of an organism, including quantitative and qualitative changes, the latter emerging with the formation of new structures and functions.

The view of development would not be complete without including the role and nature of experience. According to Gottlieb (1976), one may distinguish three distinct roles of experience in the development of behavior:

1. Experience can *maintain* or *preserve* behavioral states.

2. Experience can *facilitate* the development by accelerating its rate without changing its course or by increasing the terminal level of proficiency achieved.

3. Experience can *induce* new forms of behavior which will directly reflect the configuration of the stimulus event.

Gottlieb concludes from a review of the literature that there is evidence for the roles of maintaining and facilitating experience, but that at the moment there is no evidence for the role of inducing experience. This issue might have to do with sensitive or critical periods in development, known from research with animals, where new kinds of behavior are induced. The only behavior in children that could be related to this issue is the development of social bonds and attachment in infants.

Research Fields and Strategies in Developmental Psychopathology

In the following section, I would like to refer to some research fields and strategies in developmental psychopathology that seem important to me and promising for the near future.

Sex Differences and Individual Differences

There is a great amount of knowledge about sex differences in relation to psychopathological disorders and also of individual differences of general development. The sex differences concern physical state, growth, maturation, development of differential abilities such as speech and language functions, spatial abilities, and most psychopathological disorders (hyperkinetic syndrome, developmental delays, autism, aggressive and dissocial behavior, etc.).

Until puberty, all psychopathological conditions are more frequent in boys than in girls, though the boy–girl relation is very different for the various syndromes. For instance, the hyperkinetic syndrome is up to nine times more frequent in boys than in girls, whereas in autism the relation is only 2:1 or 3:1.

Though these differences are very clear and well established, we do not really know their cause. So this question is open for research, and several hypotheses have been offered:

— Some differences could have to do with a different maturation of the hemispheres in boys and girls. Histological studies of infant brains by Conel (1939–1960) gave evidence for the assumption that selected regions of the cortex are more mature in girls than in boys during the time from birth to the second year of life. A faster maturation may also apply to the left hemisphere and the language functions, which are more advanced in girls than in boys until puberty.

— Psychological and psychosocial factors could also be important for some of the above-mentioned sex differences. It is a well-established fact that socialization and education are different in boys and girls. Thus may one understand the proneness of girls toward depression during adolescence in the light of differential socialization patterns (Sroufe & Rutter, 1984).

— There could also be an interchange between biological factors such as maturation of the hemispheres and educational and psychosocial influences.

— It might also be possible that some differences between boys and girls are not in fact real differences, but rather caused by a different time pattern of maturation. In line with this hypothesis are the results published by Waber (1976, 1977), which demonstrate differences in psychological profiles between early and later maturers. Following this line, it could very well be that early acquired achievement structures could enhance future achievements, finally causing a new or a different quality of achievement structure. This hypothesis has to do with another open question, namely, the progressive development from quantitative to qualitative changes during development. Finally, one should mention that the androgenes play an important role in influencing maturation with long-lasting differences in neuropsychological functioning between early maturers and late maturers.

A very important issue concerning individual differences as well as sex differences is aggression. As to childhood aggression, biological factors are as important as psychological factors, for instance, a "deviation from usual attributional processes." According to Bobbitt and Keating (cit. in Sroufe &

Rutter, 1984), "the attributional error is a potentially dys-functional social cognitive skill that mediates aggressive activity in these boys."

For me our understanding of sex differences with respect to aggression in boys and girls would also be the key to our understanding of delinquency. This issue also leaves us with the open question of why there is so much continuity in aggression and dissocial behavior in boys.

Continuity and Change of Behavior

The second research field is that of continuity and discontinuity of behavior in children with respect to the developmental perspective. Although we know the different types of disorders—e.g., a continuous type remaining stable in childhood and diminishing toward adulthood, and a type of newly manifested disorder during adolescence—the cause for these different types remains unknown. Further on, the continuity of psychopathological entities from childhood to adulthood depends also (1) on the research strategy (e.g., follow-up, follow-back study), (2) the sources of information (personal investigation, interview, records, questionnaires), (3) the type of sample (clinical populations, general populations), (4) the type of disorder (neurosis, conduct disorder), (5) the outcome variables, and (6) the diagnostic criteria (Garber, 1984).

With respect to the continuity issue, those children belonging to a certain diagnostic category from the continuity type are especially interesting if they are able to stop the behavior in question on the way to adulthood.

In our delinquency study, we were able to demonstrate that positive life events (successful professional career, friends, confidence in an adult person) were associated with stopping a delinquent career (Remschmidt et al., 1984). In relation to this issue, the concept of "turning points during the individual life course" could be useful. Nevertheless, here too it has yet to be demonstrated *why* there is continuity in some children and not in others.

Risk Research

Risk research has been one of the most important issues in developmental psychopathology during the last two decades.

Within the prospective longitudinal approach, different developmental courses of children at risk were studied and compared with matched control groups. The most interesting question in this context is the development of those subjects at risk who do and do not develop the disorder in question (Garmezy, 1974; Garmezy et al., 1984; John et al., 1982; Robins, 1978).

This approach gives us not only a better understanding of the effect of risk factors, but also new insights into the process of development as such. Finally, and this is in my view the most important issue, from this study we can come to conclusions for primary prevention, which is a nearly completely unsolved problem at the moment. In this context, the following open research questions emerge:

1. What causes are at work in facilitating the manifestation of disorders in children at risk?

2. Which risk factors are most important and how do they interact with each other and with different other influences during the course of development?

3. Which influences stop the continuation of a disorder or a behavior pattern that has been in action for a certain period of time? Examples are dissocial behavior, delinquency, different anxiety states, social phobia, and depression.

The last question can be solved only by longitudinal prospective research in groups with a different load of risk factors and compared with carefully matched control groups. One problem in this context is the natural course of several disorders, which is presently unknown.

Research on Protective Factors

Risk factors and protective factors interact during the course of individual development. At the moment, we have by far more knowledge from empirical research on risk factors as compared with protective factors. The kind and nature of protective factors may be very different. We can distinguish protective factors in the child itself (e.g., high self-esteem, favorable temperamental features), within the family (e.g., high family cohesion, good relationship between the parents), and others that have to do with the availability of favorable influences in the external system. As we all know, some protective factors exist and have been studied during the last years, for example, favorable temperament, good marital relationship of the parents, high self-esteem of the child, and belonging to the female sex, which is a protective factor against psychiatric disorders, at least until puberty. Nevertheless, many questions remain open for research:

1. What are the general mechanisms in the context of which protective factors are at work?

There are, of course, hypotheses characterized by the issues of learning, maturation, identification, self-concept, interaction, and attribution. For instance, there is evidence that early secure relationships are favorable influences for the development of a high self-esteem. The same applies to successful experiences concerning a high achievement level at early age. High self-esteem and a positive self-concept are in this sense modified according to the experiences of a child.

2. What are the coping mechanisms at the different ages and developmental stages in relation to the developmental tasks?

In my view, this issue is one of the most promising in all developmental psychopathology. Table 1 gives an overview of the potential relationship between psychopathology and developmental tasks. The study of coping mechanisms in relation to developmental tasks may lead us to a better understanding of normal developmental processes as well as of pathological ones. In the clinical field, we can learn a lot from our patients by asking and observing them during their exposition of developmental tasks. Once again, it seems most interesting if, at certain stages of development, key turning points are at work in changing the course of development and making a child more resistant in the face of adverse factors. This issue, put forward by Michael Rutter, is not yet investigated, but might be a fruitful idea for our understanding of unexpected developmental changes.

3. What is the interaction of risk factors and protective factors?

It is too simple an idea that there exists a complementary relationship between risk factors and protective factors. Both kinds of influences are not independent from children's personality, from their experience, their surroundings, and the development of their self-concept. So the study of the interaction of protective and risk factors has to control many other influences. It may also be dependent on the intensity of risk factors whether protective factors are facilitated or not.

Research on Prediction

Another important task of developmental psychopathology is to study the predictive power of specific patterns of behavioral or emotional organization within the context of general development. If we look at the huge amount of influences, issues, and problems present during the course of individual development, we could arrive at the very pessimistic conclusion that prediction will not be possible at all. Several studies (Robins, 1978; Bohman, 1978; Kohlberg et al., 1972) show that this is not the case.

Why is this so?

I think there exists a hierarchy of behavioral patterns with a very different predictive power. Successful prediction of later behavior from earlier ones depends very much on the behavior pattern that was chosen as the predictor.

The following general results can be put forward (Kohlberg et al., 1972; Sroufe & Rutter, 1984):

1. Early maladaptation predicts later maladaptation (examples: school failures, poor peer relationships, pronounced antisocial behavior, overdependency in preschool age).

2. Early competence and maturity predicts later competence.

3. Absence of problems and symptoms does *not* predict later competence or maladaptation.

4. The "strongest predictors likely will be adaptational failures defined in age-appropriate terms" (Sroufe & Rutter, 1984, p. 24).

5. There is also evidence that prediction is better when using longitudinal parameters rather than cross-sectional ones.

We could demonstrate this in a study on the predictive value of weight recovery during inpatient treatment on long-term outcome in patients with anorexia nervosa. The study was carried out in 36 patients with anorexia nervosa (age at onset: 14.5 ± 1.9 years) who had been followed-up approximately 8 years later. All of them had been treated as inpatients (duration of treatment: 156 ± 76 days). For the quality of outcome, the criteria by Morgan and Russell (1975) had been used. The most important factors predictive of a good outcome were the time until stabilization of the weight curve during inpatient treatment (more than 47 days) and a stabilized weight of at least 64% of the ideal weight, a low age at onset (under 13 years), and a high variability in weight during inpatient treatment as compared with patients who had a bad prognosis. The long-term outcome could be predicted correctly in 96% of the patients with a good prognosis and in 89% of those with a poor outcome. This was done by classification and regression trees, a program with a built-in cross-validation. The results of the cross-validation were, of course, not as good, namely, 86% for a good and intermediate prognosis, and only 44% for an unfavorable outcome (Remschmidt & Müller, 1987).

Important questions for the research in prediction may be the following ones:

1. Finding out behavior patterns that have a high predictive value on different age and developmental stages concerning the natural course of behavior and the course of behavior disorders.

2. Studies on the prediction of therapy success derived from initial variables at the beginning of therapy or from variables being characteristic for the individual, the individual's family, and the disorder. For this strategy we also have a good example from our own work using initial symptomatology and family variables as predictors of therapy success.

3. Another very interesting question is the different predictive value of behavior patterns at different ages and developmental stages. All of us know that language acquisition and intelligence is of high predictive value in infantile autism. But what are the optimal predictors in these children after they have reached the age of 6? Then other predictors are important, though they are not as efficient as the two I mentioned concerning the very early stages of development. In the case of psychiatric disorders, other predictors than during normal development are important. Nevertheless, there is a relationship between developmental tasks (as steps in normal development) and symptomatology.

Classification and Categorization of Disorders and Behavior Patterns under the Developmental Perspective

Bearing the above-mentioned research fields and issues in mind, it becomes very clear that a developmental framework for classification is essential (Garber, 1984; Sroufe & Rutter, 1984). It was a progressive step that a developmental axis was included in the ICD 9 as well as in the DSM-III. The proposals for the ICD 10 and the DSM-III-R are promising and a step forward within the developmental perspective. But I think we have to go further and include the following research problems:

1. To investigate further the validity of criteria for use with adults and to develop special criteria that are specific for childhood disorders.

2. To include the issue of continuity and discontinuity of childhood disorders into the classification systems.

3. To change the focus of classification from more limited and isolated behaviors toward patterns of adaptation. These are, of course, different on different developmental stages. A good example (and probably the only one) in this field is the classification of Mary Ainsworth concerning the scheme of infant–caregiver-attachment during early infancy (Ainsworth et al., 1978): secure attachment, anxious-avoidant attachment, and anxious-resistant attachment. It has been found that these "patterns" are stable for a longer time and have a predictive value for later emotional behavior.
Meanwhile, there exist also efforts to include such patterns of adaptation into classification systems concerning behavior in preschool age (Greenspan & Lourie, 1981; Sroufe, 1983).

4. Using the idea that not only symptoms or syndromes are important for classification, but also patterns of adaptation, the idea emerged to include into a classification system also the kind and pattern of relationships. This is a very typical and important issue in developmental psychopathology, because relationships are clearly dependent on age and developmental stage.
We are just at the beginning of this issue, and under the perspective of classification of relationships, old problems of psychopathology as the continuity–discontinuity dimension and the normality–abnormality dimension have to be seen in a new light.

5. When taking up these new issues, it is at the same time important to go further on in the development of empirically derived classification systems and taxonomies. I would like to mention in this context the proposal of Tom Achenbach, which uses not only the general categories of "internalizing and externalizing behavior," but also other dimensions and especially the different sources of information (child, parents, and teachers). Thus, finally, in the classification of behavior patterns, it is very important in which context they are observed (e.g., at home, at school, or with peers). A very good example for these different perspectives is the hyperkinetic syndrome. A hyperkinetic child may not be hyperactive in a dyadic communication and situation, but very hyperactive in the classroom together with other children. So the issue of "situational context" seems to be very important. Only a few studies exist that focus the classification aspect on these contextual approaches.

Research on the Nature of the Developmental Process Itself

This theme reaches beyond the field that can be covered in this paper. Nevertheless, I would like to say a few words on this fundamental issue in developmental psychopathology. First, it has to be clear which influences have to do in a specific way with development and which do not. Second, we have to define very carefully the salient issues of developmental processes at different age periods. One example is the approach of developmental tasks, but there might be others as well. Third, it is important to differentiate between quantitative and qualitative changes during development and to focus on the relationship between or the transition from quantitative to qualitative dimensions. Piaget proposed the process of equilibration for the transition from quantitative to qualitative changes. Fourth, we should study the antecedents of psychopathology in close relation to age-defined adaptation processes. This kind of view is not static, but dynamic and includes everything discussed before. In doing this, we must be aware of the fact that development is not entirely a progressive phenomenon, but also includes regressive patterns. By this I do not mean the psychoanalytic concept of regression, but the fact that at a certain moment in development, new and progressive tendencies as well as earlier patterns of adaptation and maladaptation can be observed simultaneously, without the necessity of falling back on an earlier developmental stage, as proposed by psycho-analysts.

Finally, for normal and abnormal development, the concept of turning points seems to be important and worthy of further study. In summarizing the research notions on the nature of the developmental process itself, it is necessary to have a relatively universal model or theory of development, being able to include the already mentioned issues and being suitable for theoretically guided longitudinal research.

Models in Developmental Psychopathology

All empirical sciences use models for integrating and describing complex facts or relationships. Such models have the advantage of integrating many single observations that seem to have nothing to do with each other under the headline of a comprehensive and superior idea. Models allow also derivation of new hypotheses, the experimental confirmation or rejection of which leads to a modification of the model itself. The history of science shows that the relationships between heterogeneous results and facts could first be seen at a time at which the adequate model was present. For our purposes, we need some support through mathematical theories.

Simple Models

A very simple model for explaining reactions and achievement in different fields is the relationship of simple reaction time and age.

Figure 1 shows this relationship for a group of boys with specific reading retardation, carefully matched on social class and intelligence with a normal control group. The figure shows that there is a decline in simple reaction time with age for the normal group, but not for the boys with reading retardation. So the hypothesis emerges that specific reading retardation has to do not only with special processes of reading and writing, but probably also with a more general deficit of slower information processing in general. This first model is a very simple linear regression model.

If we look at other, more specific abilities, for instance, the detection and identification of letters on a computer screen, for the same groups, we get the model shown in Figure 2. It shows

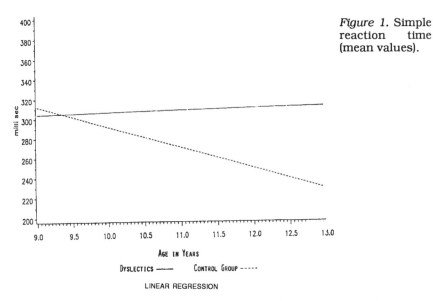

Figure 1. Simple reaction time (mean values).

a nearly linear relationship between the number of correct identifications and age for the control group, but a curvi-linear relationship for the boys with specific reading retardation. The maximum of the achievement in this task is already reached in the dyslexic boys at the age of 11.5, but not in the normal control group.

If we look at a simple concentration task in relation to age, we find a very similar picture (Figure 3), showing that the

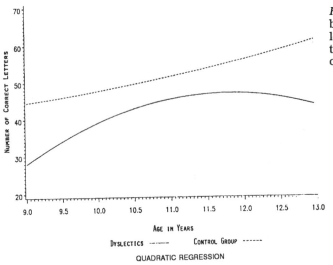

Figure 2. Number of correct letters in a letter-identificati on test.

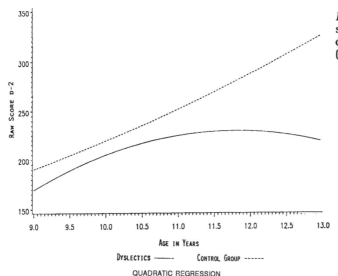

Figure 3. Raw scores in a concentration task (d2-Test).

control group can be characterized by a linear regression-type model, whereas the dyslexic boys reach the ceiling of their concentration achievement between 11.5 and 12 years, symbolized by a curvi-linear relationship (polynoma 2nd grade).

More Complex Models

Looking through the literature on models that could be useful for developmental psychopathology, I found the studies of Norman Garmezy extremely interesting (Garmezy, 1973, 1975, 1981; Garmezy et al., 1984). The studies of Garmezy and his group focus on risk, competence, and protective factors.

A simple model from the Garmezy studies is shown in Figure 4, which shows the connection between achievement, stress, and IQ (competence). It demonstrates that a high intellectual level guarantees a high achievement level under the conditions of low and also high stress. This does not apply to a lower intelligence level.

Garmezy also proposed more complex models for the relationship between competence (C) and adaptation (A).

Figure 5 shows the first complex model, which Garmezy called the "compensatory model."

1. The Compensatory Model

$$C = D + B_1A + B_2S$$

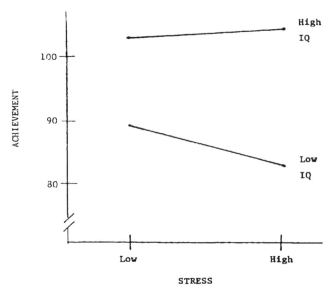

Figure 4. Interaction of stress (LEQ scores) and IQ with respect to achievement (PIAT scores).

The compensatory model shows a linear relationship between adaptation and stress. "Stress factors and personal attributes are seen as combining additively in the prediction of competence" (Garmezy et al., 1984). This means that with adaptation being constant, competence could covary negatively with the stress level. Conversely, if we hold stress (S) constant, competence (C) covaries with the strength of the adaptive possi-

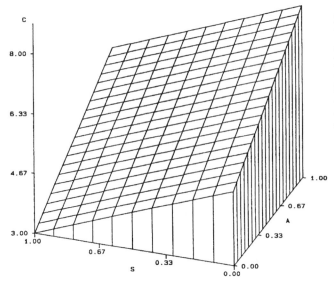

Figure 5. Compensatory model (model 1).
$C = D + B_1A + B_2S$
e.g., $C = 5 + 3A - 2S$
S = stress, A = adaptability, C = competence

bilities (A). This model is a simple linear regression model, and there is evidence for the validity of this model from the studies of Garmezy and his group.

2. The Challenge Model (Figure 6)

The "challenge model" can be symbolized by the following equation:
$$C = D + B_1A + B_2S + B_3S^2$$
The difference between model 1 and model 2 is that there is a square relationship between competence and stress instead of a linear one (as symbolized in model 1). The dependency on adaptability (A) is the same as in model 1. And as in model 1, there is no interaction effect between S and A. Changing A, while keeping S constant, results in a change in competence (C). That means that, with growing stress, competence grows in a curvi-linear way, the amount of competence being dependent on adaptability (A).

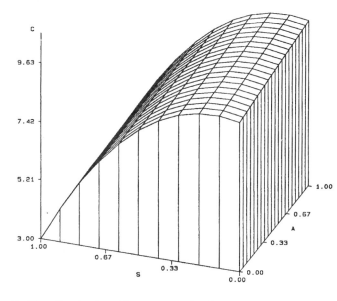

Figure 6. Challenge model (model 2). $C = D + B_1A + B_2S + B_3S^2$ e.g., $C = 8.5 + A + 2S - 7.5S^2$ S = stress, A = adaptability, C = competence

3. The Protective Factor Model (Immunity vs Vulnerability Model) (Figure 7)

This model can be symbolized by the equation:
$$C = D + B_1A + (B_2 + B_3A)S$$

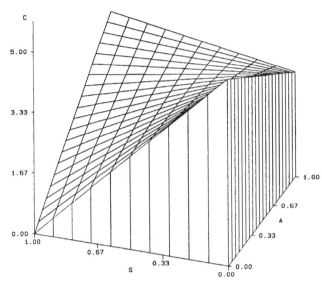

Figure 7. Protective factor model (model 3).
$C = D + B_1A + (B_2 + B_3A)S$
e.g., $C = 5 - 2A + (6A - 5)S$
S = stress, A = adaptability, C = competence

Compared with model 1 and model 2, this model includes also interactional influences. If A is constant, an increase in stress to the amount of one unit causes a change of competence by §$B_2 + B_3A$ units.

4. The Integrated Compensatory Challenge and Protective Factor Model (Figure 8)

$$C = D + B_1A + (B_2 + B_3)S + (B_4 + B_5A)S^2$$

We derived this model on the basis of the three models proposed by Garmezy et al. (1984). This new model includes the three already mentioned models in the follow way:
If $B_3 = B_4 = B_5 = 0$, model 1 results.
If $B_3 = B_5 = 0$, model 2 results.
If $B_4 = B_5 = 0$, model 3 results.
The curves of C as a function of S by keeping S constant are of the same type as in model 2 (square dependency between C and S). But as in model 3, interactions between S and A are possible, which means that the shape of the parabolic functions as well is a function of A (adaptability). The example in Figure 8 shows for A = 1 an increase of competence with growing stress up to a maximum, and then a decline of competence if stress is growing too much. For A = 0, however, the competence decreases with growing stress, even if the amount of stress is small.

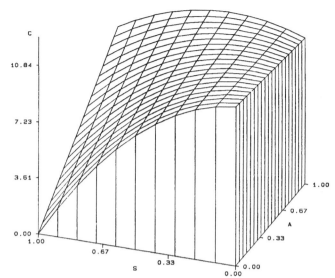

Figure 8. General model (contains models 1 to 3 as special cases).
$$C = D + B_1A + (B_2 + B_3A)S - (B_4 + B_5A)S^2$$
e.g., $C = 10 - 0.2A + (6A-1)S - (9-3A)S^2$
S = stress, A = adaptability, C = Competence.

These models are not academic games, but illustrations of the complexity of the relationship between competence, stress, and adaptability. It is possible to derive hypotheses from these models for future investigations in the field of developmental psychopathology.

The last model is really an integrative one, because it includes all the other, simpler models. The following assumptions could be formulated, bearing the last model in mind:

1. The different models could emerge in different stages of the individual development of a child.

2. It could very well be that all or some models emerge simultaneously during a certain phase of development.

3. Use of models 1, 2, or 3 could depend on the developmental level as well as the situation in which the child actually is.

4. There could very well be a dominance of using a special model or a hierarchically organized series of models as a personal and individual style of coping.

5. Finally, in the case of psychiatric disturbances, there could be a quantitatively or qualitatively different pattern of model use.

Conclusions

There have been many attempts to include the developmental perspective in the field of psychopathology in childhood. Developmental psychopathology is a relatively new field in research and is a truly integrative discipline. Important research fields include sex differences and individual differences, the issue of continuity and change of behavior, risk research, research on protective factors, on prediction, on classification, and on the nature of the developmental process itself.

Finally, it seems important to integrate and structure the existent knowledge in terms of age- and developmental-stage-related models that allow derivation of new hypotheses for the very complex process of individual development within the context of family and other components of the external system. The integrative character of developmental psychopathology requires a close collaboration of researchers of different disciplines.

References

Achenbach, T. (1974; 2nd ed. 1982). *Developmental psychopathology.* New York: Ronald.

Ainsworth, M., Blehar, M., Waters, E., & Wall, S. (1978). *Patterns of attachment.* Hillsdale, NJ: Erlbaum.

Bohman, M. (1978). Some genetic aspects of alcoholism and criminality. A population study of adoptees. *Archives of General Psychiatry, 35,* 269–276.

Bohman, M. (1980). *Adoptivkinder und ihre Familien.* Göttingen: Vandenhoeck & Ruprecht.

Cicchetti, D. (1984). The emergence of developmental psychopathology. *Child Development, 55,* 1–7.

Conel, J. (1939–1960). *The postnatal development of the human cerebral cortex, Vols. I–IV.* Cambridge, MA: Harvard University Press.

Eisenberg, L. (1977). Development as a unifying concept in psychiatry. *British Journal of Psychiatry, 131,* 225–237.

Emminghaus, H. (1887). *Die psychischen Störungen des Kindesalters.* Tübingen: Laupp.

Feldner, J. (1955). *Entwicklungspsychiatrie des Kindes.* Vienna: Springer-Verlag.

Garber, J. (1984). Classification of childhood psychopathology: A developmental perspective. *Child Development, 55*, 30–48.

Garmezy, N. (1973). Competence and adaptation in adult schizophrenic patients and children at risk. In S. R. Dean (Ed.), *Schizophrenia: The first ten Dean-Award Lectures*. New York: MSS Information Corporation.

Garmezy, N. (1974). Children at risk: The search for the antecedents of schizophrenia. I. Conceptual models and research methods. *Schizophrenia Bulletin, 8*, 14–90.

Garmezy, N. (1975). The experimental study of children vulnerable to psychopathology. In A. Davids (Ed.), *Child personality and psychopathology, Vol. 2*. New York: Wiley.

Garmezy, N. (1981). Children under stress: Perspectives on antecedents and correlates of vulnerability and resistance to psychopathology. In A. I. Rabin, J. Aronoff, A. M. Barclay, & R. A. Zucker (Eds.), *Further explorations in personality*. New York: Wiley.

Garmezy, N., Masten, A. S., & Tellegen, A. (1984). The study of stress and competence in children: A building block for developmental psychopathology. *Child Development, 55*, 97–111.

Gottlieb, G. (1976). The roles of experience in the development of behavior and the nervous system. In G. Gottlieb (Ed.), *Studies in the development of behavior and the nervous system, Vol. 3*. New York: Academic Press.

Greenspan, S., & Lourie, R. S. (1981). Developmental structuralist approach to the classification of adaptive and pathologic personality organizations: Infancy and early childhood. *American Journal of Psychiatry, 138*, 725–735.

Homburger, A. (1926). *Vorlesungen über die Psychopathologie des Kindesalters*. Berlin-Heidelberg: Springer-Verlag.

John, R., Mednick, S., & Schulsinger, F. (1982). Teacher reports as a predictor of schizophrenia and borderline schizophrenia: A bayesian decision analysis. *Journal of Abnormal Psychology, 91*, 399–413.

Kanner, L. (1935). *Child psychiatry*. Oxford: Blackwell.

Kohlberg, L., Lacrosse, J., & Ricks, D. (1972). The predictability of adult mental health from childhood behavior. In B. Wolman (Ed.), *Manual of child psychopathology*. New York: McGraw-Hill.

Morgan, H. G., & Russell, G. F. M. (1975). The value of family background and clinical features as predictors of long-term outcome in anorexia nervosa: 4-year follow-up of 41 patients. *Psychological Medicine, 5*, 355–371.

Remschmidt, H., Höhner, G., & Walter, R. (1984). Kinderdelinquenz und Frühkriminalität. In H. Göppinger & R. Vossen (Eds.), *Humangenetik und Kriminologie. Kinderdelinquenz und Frühkriminalität.* (Kriminologische Gegenwartsfragen, Bd. 16.) Stuttgart: Enke.

Remschmidt, H., & Müller, H. G. (1987). Stationäre Gewichts-Ausgangsdaten und Langzeitprognose der Anorexia nervosa. *Zeitschrift für Kinder- und Jugendpsychiatrie, 15,* 327–341.

Robins, L. (1978). Sturdy childhood predictors of adult antisocial behavior: Replications from longitudinal studies. *Psychological Medicine, 8,* 611–622.

Rolf, J., & Read, P. B. (1984). Programs advancing developmental psychopathology. *Child Development, 55,* 8–16.

Rutter, M. (1980). *Developmental psychiatry.* London: Heinemann.

Sroufe, L. A. (1983). Infant–caregiver attachment and patterns of adaptation in pre-school: The roots of maladaptation and competence. In M. Perlmutter (Ed.), *Minnesota symposia in child psychology, Vol. 16.* Hillsdale, NJ: Erlbaum.

Sroufe, L. A., & Rutter, M. (1984). The domain of developmental psychopathology. *Child Development, 55,* 17–29.

Tramer, M. (1941). *Lehrbuch der allgemeinen Kinderpsychiatrie.* Basel: Schwabe.

Waber, D. P. (1976). Sex differences in cognition: A function of maturational rate? *Science, 192,* 572–574.

Waber, D. P. (1977). Sex differences in mental abilities, hemispheric lateralization and the rate of physical growth at adolescence. *Developmental Psychology, 13,* 29–38.

Information Processing as a Theoretical Framework for Child and Adolescent Psychiatry

Rick E. Ingram

The information-processing paradigm has been extremely beneficial in the study of adult psychopathology (see Ingram, 1986). While not employed as frequently in childhood and adolescent psychopathology, it has a good deal to offer these areas as well. The present paper has several goals. First, the information-processing paradigm is broadly defined. Second, after defining information processing, some of the advantages of an information-processing perspective are described. Third, a more specific information-processing-based theoretical framework that has some promise for integrating theory and data on adult psychopathology as well as child and adolescent psychopathology is presented. And finally, several suggestions are offered as to how adoption of an information-processing perspective can guide research efforts in psychopathology. It should be noted that discussion is focused on psychopathology in general rather than on child and adolescent psychopathology in particular. While there are certainly some issues that are unique to child and adolescent disorders, the information-processing paradigm is useful for describing important aspects of any level of disordered behavior.

General Definitions of Information Processing

There are many important levels of analysis from which childhood and adolescent disorders can be viewed. The information-processing paradigm is concerned explicitly with the *cognitive* level of analysis. The information-processing paradigm derives from work in the experimental analysis of cognition. For approximately the past 25 years, experimental cognitive psychologists have been explicitly concerned with developing and empirically testing models that describe the basic nature of human cognition. Such work, however, cannot proceed in a theoretical vacuum; a conceptual paradigm is necessary to guide both the development of models and methodologies to test these models. While there are a variety of different ways of conceptualizing cognition, the dominant conceptual paradigm in cognitive psychology is that of information processing.

The information-processing paradigm initially started with an analogy to computers and suggested that, like a computer, the human being can be viewed as an information-processing system. Without taking this metaphor too far, an information-processing perspective assumes that thinking, behavior, and emotion can be understood in terms of how people process both environmental and internal information; specifically, how information is selected for processing, how it is encoded, transformed, retrieved, and otherwise manipulated. At the level of individual behavior, the information-processing paradigm is concerned with understanding the cognitive structures responsible for how people perceive—and sometimes distort—their views of themselves, others, and the world in general. This paradigm is thus concerned with the structures and operations within the cognitive system, and in the case of clinical information processing, how these structures relate to dysfunctional affect, cognition, and behavior. Understanding these structures and operations thus has implications for the conceptualization, assessment, and treatment of psychopathology (Ingram & Kendall, 1986).

There are two additional points that should help clarify the information-processing perspective further. First, the information-processing paradigm is *not* a particular model or theory; rather, information processing refers to a broad conceptual paradigm that provides a common set of assumptions for a variety of *different* cognitive theories, models, and constructs. As Anderson and Bower (1973) have aptly noted, the information-processing approach represents a "methodology for theorizing" rather than a theory per se. Thus, within the information-processing paradigm, there are a variety of theories that have been advanced to describe how individuals process information. While these theories share the common assumption that examining the way in which information is processed as well as the mechanisms responsible for this processing is a useful way to understand the functioning of individuals, they generally differ with regard to the specific theoretical constructs employed, their level of analysis, the type, degree, and scope of problems addressed, and the empirical data that are considered relevant for the particular problem. The information-processing paradigm is thus much more than a single model of cognition; it represents a broad perspective on cognition.

The second point is that there are viable alternative ways of viewing cognition. One example might be neuropsychological perspectives on cognitive functioning. As such, neuropsychology is typically concerned with elucidating brain-behavior relationships; specifically, with localizing deficits in the central nervous system, determining how these deficits are related to the functional behavior of individuals, and clinically by providing remediation strategies for these deficits. While there is certainly some overlap between neuropsychological and information-processing perspectives, the key assumptions of these approaches are different. Moreover, the utility of these approaches vary depending upon the clinical population at hand. For children and adolescents with clear evidence of central nervous system deficits or injury, that is, where there is organic involvement, neuropsychological approaches are clearly the most relevant paradigm, since they focus on brain functions. Alternatively, for the large number of children and adolescents in whom difficulties are functional rather than structural— where the "hardware" of the child's cognitive system is intact— information-processing approaches may be more relevant. Thus, while other cognitive perspectives certainly can be and are useful, the focus here is on the utility of information processing as a theoretical framework.

Advantages of an Information-Processing Perspective

There are a variety of advantages in considering an information-processing perspective as a theoretical framework. In particular, adoption of an information-processing view provides access to a diverse body of work that has accumulated in the experimental analysis of cognition. As such, information processing allows us to draw on the cognitive theory and data of basic cognition to be applied specifically to child and adolescent psychiatry in order to generate and organize data, guide conceptualization and theory, facilitate experimentally based prediction, and ultimately to provide insights into the conceptualizations, assessment, and treatment of childhood and adolescent psychopathology.

Theoretical Constructs

In addition to these general benefits, there are several specific areas of benefit. One has to do with theoretical constructs. Within information-processing approaches, numerous theoretical constructs have been developed to guide conceptualization and empirical research on cognition. To illustrate the potential of these constructs for increasing our understanding of disordered functioning, a very brief example from adult psychopathology is relevant, viz. Beck's (1967) cognitive model of depression. In attempting to account for his clinical observations of the symptoms and characteristics of depression, Beck first invoked the notion of cognitive schemes (representing an information-processing theoretical construct) and explained depression in terms of "faulty patterns of information processing." That is, individuals are proposed to become depressed because they negatively distort the information they process about themselves, their world, and their future. Since that time, Beck's model has generated an enormous amount of research and subsequent theory. Moreover, it has also led directly to the development of a treatment strategy based directly on the information-processing model—a treatment commonly referred to as "cognitive therapy of depression" (Beck et al., 1979). Empirical data generated by a number of different investigators and accumulating since 1977 have consistently shown that this therapeutic approach is effective not only for treating depression, but also for preventing relapse. This is one concrete example of how constructs adopted from information processing can be useful not only in conceptualizing psychopathology, but in developing effective treatment strategies as well.

Empirical Methodologies

A second advantage of an information-processing perspective derives from examination of the empirical methodologies typically employed in this paradigm. A fundamental aspect of information processing is an empirical methodology developed explicitly to assess the parameters of cognitive variables. To take yet another example from adult psychopathology, Saccuzzo and colleagues (see Saccuzzo, 1986) have employed what is known as a "backward masking" technology based on information processing which requires subjects to identify briefly presented target stimuli under several varying conditions. By examining the speed and accuracy with which schizophrenic subjects are able to perform this task, Saccuzzo has been able to generate several inferences concerning the attentional deficits usually found in schizophrenia. Such inferences, and the theoretical models of attentional deficits in schizophrenia based on these inferences, would not have been possible without employing an information-processing perspective as a theoretical framework.

Information-Processing Findings

A final advantage of the information-processing paradigm has to do with the findings generated in experimental cognitive psychology, many of which are potentially useful for clinical researchers. Turning once again to the area of adult depression, several experimental findings concerning basic memory processes have been extremely helpful in disentangling the specific types of memory distortions that contribute to depressive symptomatology. In particular, these findings in basic cognitive psychology have led to data showing that depressed individuals evidence an oversensitivity to negative-content information, which appears to contribute to their depression (see Ingram & Reed, 1986). Again, such results would not have been possible without an appreciation of an information-processing approach to human behavior.

Thus far, the attempt has been made to give a broad definition of the information-processing paradigm and to provide some examples of how information processing can serve as a useful theoretical framework for guiding research efforts. Although the examples provided have all been in the realm of adult psychopathology, such examples can also be applied to child and adolescent psychopathology. I would like to turn now to a discussion of a more specific information-processing-based model that has some promise for integrating several different levels of cognitive analysis into a more comprehensive framework for understanding the role of cognitive variables in both adult and childhood psychopathology.

The Meta-Construct Model of Psychopathology

As clinical research has become increasingly more cognitive in its orientation, an almost overwhelmingly large number of cognitive constructs have been proposed to account for various aspects of psychopathology. Because there are so many constructs, at present it is not clear which of these many constructs, or sets of constructs, capture the essential elements of a given disorder. Extant concepts of cognitive factors span a wide range of different "types" of cognition and levels of cognitive analysis. In depression, for example, depression-linked differences have been found in cognitive variables ranging from specific information-retrieval processes to generalized dysfunctional belief systems. Advances in our understanding of psychopathology requires an integration of these different cognitive variables. The framework to be described, called the *meta-construct model of psychopathology* (Ingram, 1988; Ingram & Wisnicki, in press) is a generalized information-processing model of psychopathology aimed at describing and classifying various levels of cognitive analysis. The model incorporates two theoretical approaches to the description of different psychological functioning: a *cognitive taxonomy* that denotes various categories of cognitive constructs proposed to describe maladaptive functioning (Ingram, 1983; Ingram & Kendall, 1986, 1987; Kendall, 1985; see also Goldfried & Robins, 1983; Hammen, 1981; Hollon & Kriss, 1984; Marzillier, 1980; Turk & Speers, 1983); and a *components models of psychopathology* that seeks to examine the cognitive features that are unique to a particular disorder as well as those that appear to be generalized across different disorders (Ingram & Kendall, 1987; Kendall & Ingram, 1987). The meta-construct model proposes a structure for organizing both the taxonomy and the components model into broad conceptual categories that encompass both similar and different information-processing features.

Cognitive Taxonomy Elements

In an effort to organize the numerous kinds of cognitive constructs that have been proposed to characterize psychopathology, we have suggested a cognitive taxonomy to describe the general categories into which these constructs fall. These categories consists of cognitive *structural, propositional, oper-*

ational, and *product* variables. While these categories are proposed to be distinct in a conceptual sense, constructs within each category operate jointly to produce what is typically referred to as cognition.

Cognitive Structural Constructs

Structural concepts refer broadly to the "architecture" of the cognitive system in that these variables describe mechanisms encompassing how information is stored and organized. Concepts such as short- and long-term memory are noteworthy examples of variables that focus upon the structural aspects of information processing. Thus, for example, information-processing models of dysfunction that view deficiencies in long-term memory as the key to the disorder would be focusing on cognitive structural variables.

Cognitive Propositional Constructs

Structural mechanisms are by definition "contentless"; propositions refer to the content of information that is stored and organized within a structure. Episodic and semantic knowledge represent illustrations of propositional variables. It should be noted that because this category describes the stored content of the cognitive system, it could easily be labeled as cognitive content. Since "content" is used in different ways to describe different phenomena (e.g., the content of self-statements, the content of beliefs, etc.), the term "propositions" was chosen to decrease ambiguity between classes of cognitive variables.

Cognitive Operational Constructs

Operations consist of the processes by which the system works. Some examples of cognitive operations variables include information encoding, retrieval, and attentional processes.

Cognitive Product Constructs

Products are defined as the end result of the operation of the cognitive system to process information; these are the cognitions or thoughts that the individual experiences as a result of the interaction of incoming information with cognitive structures, propositions, and operations. Examples include constructs such as attributions or cognitive self-statements. Since an attribution is an individual's causal explanation of a prior behavioral event, it results from (is a product of) cognitive processing of related content. Thus, we suggest that most of the major cognitive constructs proposed by theories of psychopathology will fall into one of these categories.

Components Model of Psychopathology

Partitioning the Variance in Psychopathology

It is unrealistic to assume that all or most cognitive variables are unique to a particular psychological disorder. We suggest that a useful metaphor for understanding how these variables relate to different disorders is to employ a model that views the variance in psychopathology analogously to the manner in which variance is conceptualized in experimental research (Ingram & Kendall, 1987). Specifically, we propose that the variance in psychopathology can be conceptually "partitioned" in much the same way as experimental variance is partitioned by an ANOVA. Hence, the ultimate symptomatic expression of a disorder is a function of several converging and identifiable sources of variance. For example, a two-way ANOVA would partition an experimental result into components represented as: Effect = A + B + AB + E, where A equals the unique variance due to the first factor, B equals the unique variance due to the second factor, AB equals the common or shared variance resulting from the interaction of the factors, and E represents the error variance. In a similar fashion, the expression of a particular psychopathology can be conceptualized as the result of the confluence of "critical psychopathological features," "common psychopathological features," and unpredictable error variance.

Critical Features

These features represent variance that is uniquely characteristic of a particular disorder and thus describe variables specific to a given psychopathology. Hence, these features are defined as those that not only differentiate disorder from non-disorder, but also that differentiate one disorder from another.

Common Features

In contrast to critical psychopathological features, common features are those that are generally characteristic of all or most disorders and are therefore conceptualized as common or shared psychopathological variance. While these features do not differentiate particular disorders, they are defined as differentiating disorder from non-disorder. That is, while common features are not unique to a given disorder, they are "unique" to psychopathology in general and thus broadly separate adaptive from maladaptive functioning.

Error Variance

Finally, error variance represents the unpredictable variance in psychopathology arising from nonsystematic factors. While the majority of variance in the expression of psychopathology can most likely be accounted for by critical and common features, the precise symptoms and characteristics of the disorder will also be influenced to some degree by the factors unique to the particular person involved. However, since error variance is by definition unpredictable, it will not be discussed further.

Interactions

In a two or higher way ANOVA model, interactions are possible between independent variables. At present we do not have an interaction term in the meta-construct model. Such interactions are theoretically possible in that certain combinations of psychopathological states may produce cognitive characteristics that are sufficiently different from either state alone. At present, however, there are insufficient empirical data to speculate on how various interactions of different disorders differ from either disorder alone.

It is also important to note that the ANOVA metaphor should not be taken too literally by suggesting that all components of the ANOVA must be represented in the corresponding psychopathology conceptual model (such as interactions). That is, the ANOVA model is simply a useful analogy for thinking about how psychopathological variance can be broken down into specific and nonspecific aspects. Any other statistical procedure partitioning sources of variance (e.g., multiple regression, factor analysis) would serve just as well as a model for separating elements of psychopathology into conceptually interesting segments.

Together, the cognitive taxonomy model and the cognitive components approach can be combined into the meta-construct model as a way of integratively classifying cognitive features in various disorders. What this model suggests is a framework for classifying various disorders in terms of the structural, propositional, operational, and products variables that characterize the disorder and the separation of each of these variables into critical (or unique) and common features. For different disorders the critical features at each level of analysis will be very different, while the common features should look very similar. The model is thus set up to help conceptually classify the variety of cognitive features that can be studied in different disorders.

The meta-construct model can be used to illustrate how information-processing approaches can be used to understand any level of psychopathology, including childhood and adolescent psychopathology. From a *descriptive psychopathology* standpoint, for example, it is possible to examine the cognitive similarities and differences among different disorders, i.e., the meta-construct model suggests that various disorders are characterized by cognitive variables that are unique to the particular disorder as well as those that are common to a number of disorders. Employing this model as a guiding framework suggests two things for researchers. First, that any cognitive or information-processing assessment must be broad-spectrum assessment that examines a number of different variables at different cognitive levels. Otherwise, important data as to the *pattern* of cognitive similarities and differences will be missed if only single variables are assessed, thus leading to potentially misleading conclusions. Second, generating comparative data across different child and adolescent disorders within the context of an integrative cognitive framework allows for the potential to discover cognitive variables that are unique to particular disorders. Consequently, these unique variables may prove to be the critical cognitive processes that determine the disorder or characteristics of the disorder. Thus, by recommending broad cognitive assessment over different psychopathologies, the information-processing paradigm provides useful frameworks for basic descriptive investigations into the cognitive mechanisms of childhood and adolescent psychiatric disorders.

The information-processing paradigm also provides frameworks for examining *vulnerability* factors for disorder. In this vein, a number of investigators have begun to examine the information-processing characteristics of children and families that are vulnerable to disorder. Ian Gotlib in Canada and Constance Hammen in the United States, for example, are starting to look at the interactions of depressed mothers and their children in longitudinal experiments in order to examine information-processing patterns early on that may predict eventual childhood disorder. Similarly, several investigators have assessed information processing in the families of schizophrenics to see if there are early signs of dysfunctional information processing that might predict the onset of schizophrenia. Thus, information-processing paradigms have been used to examine both how dysfunctional families may affect the cognitive characteristics of children who might later become dysfunctional as well as to look at dysfunctional families that may predispose children to become dysfunctional adults. It seems clear that research guided by general information-processing assumptions as well as by specific information-processing models such as the meta-construct model offer the potential to tell us a great deal about how and why disordered children and adolescents are different from normal children and adolescents.

In conclusion, the information-processing paradigm has great promise as a guiding theoretical framework for child and adolescent psychiatry. It is always important to note, however, that there are many important levels of analysis. Ultimately, any comprehensive understanding of childhood and adolescent psychiatric disorders will come from data and theories that integrate cognitive, behavioral, social, biological, and genetic explanations of behavior. To the extent that the cognitive level of analysis is an important one, the information-processing paradigm can help us to understand this level.

References

Anderson, J. R., & Bower, G. H. (1973). *Human associative memory.* Washington: Erlbaum.

Beck, A. T. (1967). *Depression: Clinical, theoretical, and experimental aspects.* New York: Hoeber.

Beck, A. T., Rush, A. J., Shaw, B. F., & Emery, G. (1979). *Cognitive therapy of depression.* New York: Guilford Press.

Goldfried, M. R., & Robins, C. (1983). Self-schema, cognitive bias, and the processing of therapeutic experiences. In P. C. Kendall (Ed.), *Advances in cognitive-behavioral research and therapy, Vol. 2* (pp. 33–80). New York: Academic Press.

Hammen, C. L. (1981). Assessment: A clinical and cognitive emphasis. In L. P. Rehm (Ed.), *Behavior therapy for depression: Present status and future direction* (pp. 255–277). Orlando, FL: Academic Press.

Hollon, S. D., & Kriss, M. (1984). Cognitive factors in clinical research and practice. *Clinical Psychology Review, 4,* 35–76.

Ingram, R. E. (1983). Content and process distinctions in depressive self-schemata. In L. B. Alloy (Chair), *Depression and schemata.* Symposium presented at the meeting of the American Psychological Association, Anaheim, CA.

Ingram, R. E. (Ed.) (1986). *Information processing approaches to clinical psychology.* Orlando, FL: Academic Press.

Ingram, R. E. (1988). *Self-focused attention in clinical disorders: Review and a conceptual model.* Manuscript submitted for publication.

Ingram, R. E., & Kendall, P. C. (1986). Cognitive clinical psychology: Implications of an information processing perspective. In R. E. Ingram (Ed.), *Information processing approaches to clinical psychology* (pp. 3–21). Orlando, FL: Academic Press.

Ingram, R. E., & Kendall, P. C. (1987). The cognitive side of anxiety. *Cognitive Theory and Research, 11,* 523–536.

Ingram, R. E., & Reed, M. (1986). Information encoding and retrieval processes in depression: Findings, issues, and future directions. In R. E. Ingram (Ed.), *Information processing approaches to clinical psychology.* Orlando, FL: Academic Press.

Ingram, R. E., & Wisnicki, K. S. (in press). Cognition in depression. In P. Magaro & M. Johnson (Eds.), *Annual review of psychopathology.* JAI Press.

Kendall, P. C. (1985). Toward a cognitive-behavioral model of child psychopathology and a critique of related interventions. *Journal of Abnormal Child Psychology, 13,* 357–372.

Kendall, P. C., & Ingram, R. E. (1987). The future for cognitive assessment of anxiety: Let's get specific. In L. Michelson & L. M. Ascher (Eds.), *Anxiety and stress disorders: Cognitive-behavioral assessment and treatment* (pp. 89–104). New York: Guilford Press.

Marzillier, J. S. (1980). Cognitive therapy and behavioural practice. *Behaviour Research and Therapy, 18,* 249–288.

Saccuzzo, D. P. (1986). An information processing interpretation of theory and research in depression. In R. E. Ingram (Ed.), *Information processing approaches to clinical psychology.* Orlando, FL: Academic Press.

Turk, D. C., & Speers, M. A. (1983). Cognitive schemata and cognitive processes in cognitive behavioral interventions: Going beyond the information given. In P. C. Kendall (Ed.), *Advances in cognitive-behavioral research and therapy, Vol. 2* (pp. 1–32). New York: Academic Press.

Structural Models and Longitudinal Data in Research on Risk Factors in Adolescent Development*

Rainer K. Silbereisen

Developmental psychopathology is conceived as an interdisciplinary approach toward a better understanding of the interplay between adaptation and maladaptation across the life-span (Rutter & Garmezy, 1983). As with research on human development in general, investigators strive here too for explanatory analyses rather than mere descriptions of change.

In the past decade efforts toward this goal have seen a growing merge between structural modeling techniques and longitudinal research design (Rogosa, 1979; McArdle, 1988). One major reason is that repeated measurements of the same variables ease the otherwise cumbersome task of identifying cause-effect relations in non-experimental data. The development of elegant mathematical procedures and program packages such as LISREL (Jöreskog & Sörbom, 1986) provided a further impetus.

The paper deals with four issues related to the application of structural modeling in longitudinal research on risk factors in adolescent development: design, concepts of change, person-process-context models, and comparative research strategies. The aim is to show some typical problems and discuss ways to resolve them.

These issues will be illustrated by examples from the Berlin Youth Longitudinal Study that my colleagues and I have been conducting since 1981 (see Verdonik & Sherrod, 1984, for a short technical reference, and Silbereisen & Noack, in press, for representative results). The principal aim is the analysis of the role of problem behavior in normal adolescent development. Risk and protective factors within the individual, and within family, work, and leisure contexts, have been investigated in Berlin (West) and Warsaw (Poland). By 1989, one of the cohorts

* The research was supported in part by German Research Council Grants to R. K. Silbereisen (Si 296/1-1 through 6, co-investigator K. Eyferth, and Si 296/3-1). Thanks are extended to Helfried T. Albrecht for helpful comments.

(three in each city) will have been followed up once every year from ages 11 to 18.

Design

The advantages of longitudinal, multi-cohort measurements of change as compared to cross-sectional studies on age differences are well known (Nesselroade & Baltes, 1979). However, restrictions in terms of time, effort, and financial resources available limit longitudinal assessment and analysis. Furthermore, repeated measurements have their own costs in terms of attrition and carry-over effects between waves of measurements.

Convergence Method

The so-called convergence method proposed over three decades ago by Bell (1954) is a widely overlooked alternative. The method consists of making limited remeasurements of cross-sectional groups so that temporarily overlapping measurements can be used as a means of linking up between adjacent segments of a developmental function. Thus, instead of measuring adolescent self-esteem every year between ages 11 and 18, one may well use two age cohorts, 11- and 14-year-olds, and have three or four measurements per cohort in yearly intervals. The advantage in terms of subject motivation and participation, respectively, may be remarkable.

Earlier statistical approaches to this design have been criticized (Nesselroade & Baltes, 1979). Recently, McArdle et al. (1987) demonstrated how modern structural modeling techniques provide ways to analyze such cross-sequential designs. Given the cohorts overlap, the assumption of convergent age trends can be tested. Based on my own experience, the convergence approach would help to ease the implementation of longitudinal research.

Time-Lags

There is another widely overlooked problem in planning longitudinal research: Most often the length of the time intervals between measurements is legitimized for pragmatic reasons only, which may introduce serious bias into the models under scrutiny (Gollob & Reichardt, 1987). In the Berlin Youth Longitudinal Study, for instance, the sample was organized and the assessments were made within school settings. Because of organizational constraints, we could contact the adolescents only once a year. For some of the variables, this time-span may be adequate; for others, however, it may be much too long. While a variable such as self-esteem will not show much change within 12 months, less stable variables such as mood states will oscillate several times. Though variable rather than constant assessment intervals would be favorable, the only alternative is to include retrospective data within each wave of measurement. Research by Kandel (Kandel et al., 1987) using event history analysis is a case in point. In order to study the influence of transitions such as marriage or unemployment, she assessed substance use retrospectively for each three-month period.

Concepts of Change

The lack of theoretical considerations prior to empirical testing is ubiquitous. As Biddle and Marlin (1987) put it, structural equation modeling appears to be misunderstood and misused by many persons. More specifically, questions have been raised as to the specification of structural models representing processes of change.

Autoregressive Models

A case in point is the popular autoregressive model. The question is whether one should assume cross-lagged or contemporaneous effects between variables. In Figure 1, results of Galambos and Silbereisen (1987) are shown. Using path-analytic methods, we studied relations across three waves of measurement between substance use, contacts with deviant peers, and school failure.

The paths from deviant peers and substance use, respectively, to school failure cannot be read as indicating a cross-lagged effect; rather, these paths result from the fact that school failure was not measured at the first wave of measurement. In accordance with this interpretation, such effects were not present between the second and third wave. Instead, simple covariations represent the issue.

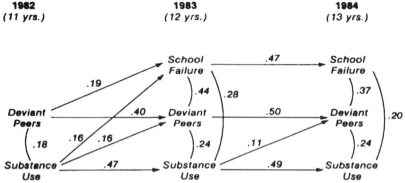

Figure 1. Path model for n = 373 adolescents (median age at first measurement: 11.5 years). Significant standardized regression coefficients and within-time correlations are shown. *Substance Use* is a combined scale of the frequency of cigarette smoking and consumption of beer or wine in the last year (wave 1: ever used). *Contacts with Deviant Peers* was measured by four items (e.g., "My friends often get into trouble with adults"). *School Failure* was assessed through two items (e.g., "My teachers think that I am a failure").(Reprinted by permission from Galambos & Silbereisen, 1987.)

What about the cross-lagged effects between substance use and deviant peers? Though we are quite sure that effects in the opposite direction can be deemed irrelevant, there is no way to guarantee that the assumption of a considerable time-lag is adequate. Rather, this is a presupposition that needs independent evidence, preferably grounded in conceptual considerations. If substance use would "go with" contacts with deviant peers, then a model assuming contemporaneous effects might be more adequate.

Further results (not reported here) demonstrated differences between age cohorts. While substance use seems to play a role in leading early adolescents to associate with deviant peers, this effect was not present in middle adolescence when most subjects had made the transition to having tried smoking and drinking.

Concerning the validity of the autoregressive model some general recommendations were made by Hertzog and Nesselroade (1987). Its application is legitimized in cases where the variables are characterized by high stability and low degree of situational and temporal specificity. Let me illustrate these principles by another example from our own research where we (Silbereisen & Reitzle, in press) discussed a model that reveals releasing ("cathartic") leisure motives as mediating factors in linking self-esteem and alcohol use. In Figure 2 the structural model is shown for a group of female adolescents.

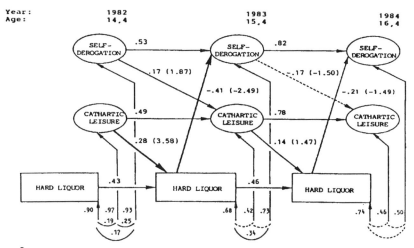

Chi²=340.54, df=285, GFI=.909, RMSR=.047

Figure 2. Structural equation model for use of beer or wine in n = 206 female adolescents. *Self-Derogation* (low self-esteem) was measured by a four-item scale (e.g., "I don't think I'm worth very much"). *Cathartic Leisure* was a scale comprised of six items. Adolescents had to indicate how likely they would be to release their frustration from a day marked by failure at school or at home by roaming about the neighborhood, playing with pinball or video machines, listening to music full blast at home, and the like. Significant (heavy solid arrows) and tentatively significant (solid arrows) standardized structural coefficients (path coefficients) among constructs are depicted (dotted arrows represent postulated but statistically irrelevant coefficients). Numbers in parentheses are T-values used in evaluating the structural coefficients. Furthermore, for each construct disturbance terms per wave are given (solid lines if significant).

The case in point is the effect of prior cathartic leisure on future use of beer or wine and its improving effect on consequent self-esteem. As we pointed out, evidence indicates a process by which problems with one's self-esteem lead to an increase in cathartic leisure orientation that, in turn, increased the risk of alcohol use. The latter, however, helped to improve the girls' self-appreciation. Interestingly enough, this chain of effects was found for females only. Furthermore, it was even somewhat clearer for hard liquor. We interpreted this as indicating differences in the gender-specific range of "optimal non-normativity" (cf. Gold & Petronio, 1980). For girls, drinking alcohol is deviant enough to attract attention by peers, but, at the same time, is normative enough in order to avoid any subsequent punishment by parents.

Concerning self-esteem and leisure motives, the autoregressive approach seems to be justified by the high stabilities. Concerning alcohol, however, this assumption is tenuous.

Discrete Events or Continuous Change

Often researchers depict the influence across time of one variable on another variable by simply characterizing it as a series of discrete events rather than a process of continuous change. In fact, this is what we did in the previous example. An alternative way of tackling this problem was recently suggested by Labouvie and Nesselroade (1988). Instead of assuming a linkage between the variables through initial differences only, additional effects are seen as resulting from differential amounts of change across time. The basic idea is depicted in Figure 3.

As can be seen, cathartic leisure (CL) and substance use (SU) are longitudinally related by way of an autoregressive model. However, terms indicating the differential amount of change across time are part of the model. Thus, cathartic leisure at year 2 (CLYR2) is assumed to be influenced by cathartic leisure and substance use of the previous year, and the change in substance use from year 1 to year 2 (SUYR2-1). Similarly, substance use at year 2 is influenced by the change in cathartic leisure (CLYR2-1). The same principles hold for the third wave of measurement (SUYR3-2 and CLYR3-2).

It is important to keep in mind that, in terms of model-fitting, one cannot differentiate between the two alternatives.

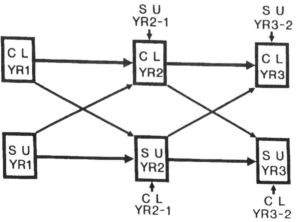

Figure 3. A three-wave (YR1, YR2, YR3) autoregressive model with cross-lagged effects is shown linking *Cathartic Leisure* (CL) and *Substance Use* (SU). Variables at waves 2 and 3 are additionally influenced by effects due to differential amount of change across time (e.g., SUYR2-1).

Person-Process-Context Models

The ultimate goal of research in developmental psychopathology is a better understanding of the processes that lead to impaired development. These processes, however, may vary among subpopulations.

In conceptual work on the ecology of human development, a similar argument was advanced. Bronfenbrenner (Bronfenbrenner & Crouter, 1983; Bronfenbrenner, 1988) propagated the idea that—contrary to common presupposition in research practice—developmental processes are not invariant across both person and context. They do not vary only in magnitude, but also in direction as a function of the interplay between the nature of the context and the character of the person. The notion of person-process-context models demands research designs that can illuminate the variability of developmental processes as a function of person and context variables (Silbereisen & Walper, 1988 a).

Concerning research on risk factors in adolescent development, studies on the effect of economic hardship on family functioning and personality development of the adolescent offspring are one of the few instances where models on complex multi-stage risk mechanisms were extensively studied. Following Elder's approach (Elder et al., 1984a, b), we investigated the impact of economic loss on adolescents' self-esteem and contranormative orientations, focusing on the mediating role of strained family relations. Using data from the Berlin Youth Longitudinal Study, Walper and Silbereisen (1987) studied families who had reported a loss in family income of at least 5–25% or more during the previous year. They were compared with income-stable families matched on socioeconomic variables, age, and sex of the adolescent child. Economic loss was shown to lead to impaired family integration and lower self-esteem among the adolescents. Lower self-esteem, in turn, mediated the effects of income loss and family integration on the adolescents' transgression proneness.

However, this was only true for families in which at least one of the parents had no high school degree. In contrast, in families with higher educational levels—that is, both parents being high school graduates—the income loss showed no significant effects on family integration and self-esteem. Thus, only the group low in parental education showed the effects known from the Great Depression in the 1930s. Educational level was used in order to assess one important aspect of the contexts in which the people live. It is meant as a proxy to the availability of resources to cope with hardships.

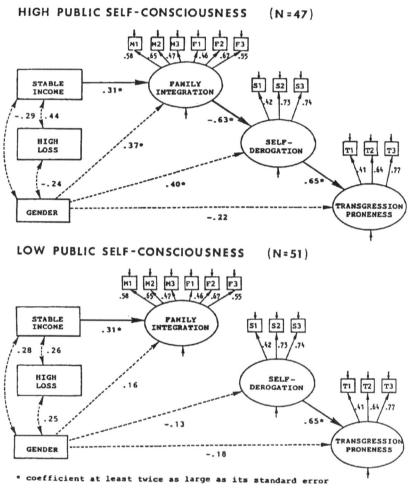

Figure 4. Structural models on the effects of economic hardship for adolescents high and low in *Public Self-Consciousness*, measured by four items like "I become curious when others talk about me." *Family Integration* (e.g., "If something needs to be done at home, everybody tries to get out of it"; inverted), *Self-Derogation* (e.g., "I don't think I'm worth very much"), and *Transgression Proneness* (e.g., "I often find the rules and laws of adults bad and don't like to follow them") are comprised of four items each. *Stable Income* contrasts no loss with loss of any kind, *High Loss* contrasts loss of 25% and more with moderate loss between 5% and 25%.

Walper and Silbereisen (1987 a, b) tried to better understand the unexpectedly weak relation between family integration and self-esteem in their earlier study. Drawing from research on public self-consciousness, we hypothesized family integration to influence only those adolescents who are highly sensitive to self-related information provided by others.

In Figure 4 the results of a structural modeling approach are shown. The design and the subjects are identical to those of the earlier study.

As shown, a mediational effect was observed only for the group high in public self-consciousness. Here, income loss—with stable income the contrast is indicated between loss of any kind and no loss—influenced self-derogation mediated by family integration. Adolescents low in public self-consciousness, however, did not reveal the links between family relations and self-esteem.

The analyses reported thus far did not utilize repeated measurements. In a recent paper (Silbereisen & Walper, 1988 b), we showed cross-lagged effects as well. For instance, transgression proneness measured in the previous year influenced family integration, which in turn influenced transgression proneness.

The group of families who had to cope with economic hardship was too small to break down further as to the interaction of context (educational level) and person variables (public self-consciousness). Furthermore, the differences between the subsamples are somewhat exaggerated by the method used. When applying multi-group comparisons as available with LISREL, the commonalities prevail.

This leads to an important caveat. In order to avoid "capitalizing on chance," sample sizes have to be large. Cross-validation using independent samples is mandatory. Furthermore, the researcher should try to find a superordinate model that fits the structures in the subsamples. Only if this attempt fails is the person-process-context approach adequate.

Comparative Research Strategies

Risk factors in adolescent development—for instance, unemployment, school drop-out, teenage pregnancy, violence, and substance use—show rather substantial differences in prevalence and quality as a function of the cultural or subcultural context. Identical labels for these phenomena should not be misunderstood as indicating similar developmental processes involved. Thus, comparative strategies, especially those inherent to cross-cultural research, are mandatory.

Timing of Maturation

A case in point are normative transitions within the school system. According to a number of studies conducted in the United States (e.g., Simmons et al., 1983), students who undergo a transition after grade 6 from a small elementary school into a larger junior high school suffer more in terms of their self-esteem than do students who remain in an elementary school setting until grade 8. This effect seemed to be especially pronounced among girls.

A plausible explanation refers to the interplay between biological and social factors. The timing of maturation seems to be crucial. In contrast to boys, girls were reported to suffer from early maturation. Their self-esteem is lower, and many react by withdrawal in achievement situations (Petersen & Crockett, 1985).

Thus, transition after grade 6 may confront early maturing girls with too many challenges to cope with at the same time. In the extreme, they may lack an "arena of comfort" that, according to Simmons et al. (1987), is the backbone of adolescent well-being. Meanwhile, new policies and programs on preventive intervention question well-established school organizational principles such as the transition from junior to senior high school. New ideas aiming at an enrichment of the middle schools have been developed (Carnegie Corporation, 1988).

In sum, research on negative effects of transitions in the school system have fueled the debate on educational reforms. However, we may ask whether the results indeed shed light on universals of adolescent development. Other countries and cultures may vary not only in the timing and quality of the transition, but also in the psychosocial impact of early maturation. In the following, I would like to exemplify the problems.

In a recent paper (Silbereisen et al., 1988), we checked the impact of early versus late maturation with a sample of girls drawn from the files of the Berlin Youth Longitudinal Study. In contrast to earlier research, we addressed the role of maturational timing within a rather complex model of the development of problem behavior in adolescence. As expected, peer rejection played a major role. Those who were rejected by their classmates had more contacts with deviant peers, showed a higher proneness for transgression, and had a lower self-esteem. For girls in middle adolescence (age 14 to 15 on average), late maturation corresponded to lower self-esteem, whereas early maturation corresponded to higher self-esteem as compared to their same-aged peers. In addition, there was a slight tendency among early maturing girls to report more contacts with deviant peers. However, early maturation did not show the adverse effects on self-esteem as expected on the basis of the U.S. studies.

Self-Esteem and School Transition

Using a sample also drawn from the Berlin Youth Longitudinal Study, the effect of the school transition on students' self-esteem was analyzed. In Berlin (West), educational tracking takes place after grade 6 as in the United States. However, tracking implies more than a mere shift in the school ecology. Students are placed into different tracks depending on earlier achievement. Furthermore, probable life prospects are still dependent on the type of school one attends. Thus, tracking has a considerable impact on the pathways of development.

Our results reveal a contrast to what one would expect from the U.S. data. In Figure 5 the results of a structural modeling approach are depicted. Self-esteem was measured in five consecutive years for grades 5 through 9 (1982–1986), using two indicators (C: willingness to change; S: self-evaluation). As the factor loadings were set equally, the measure of self-esteem can be deemed identical from year to year. As shown, the stabilities across time are quite high (highest from grades 8 to 9: .78).

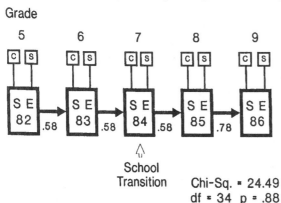

Grade

Figure 5. Structural model for n = 169 adolescents. *Self-Esteem* (SE) was measured by two sum-indicators: C refers to adolescents' willingness to change (e.g., "Sometimes I wish I were different"), S to their self-evaluation (e.g., "I don't think I'm worth very much"). The transition into different educational tracks takes place after grade 6.

School Transition   Chi-Sq. = 24.49 df = 34 p = .88

Table 1. Effects of gender and educational track on students' (low) self-esteem for grades 5 through 9.

	Grade/Year				
Effects	5/82	6/83	7/84	8/85	9/86
Gender					
Male (1)	−.15	−.07	.02	−.08	−.24*
Educational track[a]					
Low (2)	.43**	.35**	.10	−.07	.02
Medium (3)	.00	.07	.07	.10	−.12
High (4)	−.43**	−.42**	−.17	−.03	.10
Interactions					
(1) × (2)	−.09	−.16	−.24+	−.24	.05
(1) × (3)	−.09	.14	.42*	.43*	.31+
(1) × (4)	.18	.02	−.18	−.19	−.36*

Note: Regression on latent variables (low) self-esteem in 1982 through 1986 for N=169 students. Latent variables are centered with mean = 0. Thus, regression coefficients express deviation from 0 due to effects of gender, educational tracks in school, and their interactions (low = *Gesamtschule*, medium = *Realschule*, high = *Gymnasium*). Exogenous variables are effect-coded. Negative scores indicate *higher* self-esteem.
[a]Transition into different tracks takes place in grade 7. Thus, for grades 5 and 6 educational track refers to *future* track.
+ = p<.10, * = p<0.05, ** = p<0.01

The sample was broken down as to educational track for each year, including the pretracking years (using the placement that was observed following grade 6). In Table 1 the effects of gender and educational track on students' (low) self-esteem are indicated.

A main effect of gender was observed for the last wave of measurement only. In grade 9 male adolescents reported a higher self-esteem than females. In the years preceding the transition, there is a contrast between low and high tracks. Whereas future college track students show a higher self-esteem, students in the lowest track show the opposite effect. In the years following the transition, it is the male students of the middle track who report the lowest self-esteem.

Transition in school seems to imply different strains and challenges in West Germany as compared to the United States. Based on the American studies we would have expected a marked gender effect on self-esteem subsequent to the transition. Instead, no effects were found at grades 7 and 8 in the present data. Furthermore, the difference in self-esteem between students of highest and lowest tracks is lowered following the transition. In sum, our analyses reveal different processes in the two cultures: While the American system pulls boys and girls apart in respect to self-esteem, the German system provides the chance for decreasing differences in self-esteem between students of both genders following the transition in school.

The advantage of comparative strategies is obvious. Whenever we are interested in the long-term consequences of complex social structures, cross-cultural variation may be used as a quasi-experimental design. Thus, by varying the cultural background, the effects of timing and quality of transitions in the school system on personality development can be separated.

Final Remarks

Structural modeling can help to improve research on risk factors for adolescent development. However, as Baumrind (1983) put it, too many studies lack theoretical analysis prior to empirical testing. Another pitfall is the common practice to report models that were modified post hoc in order to maximize goodness-of-fit. Though this strategy requires cross-validation, replication studies are still the exception.

References

Baumrind, D. (1983). Specious causal attributions in the social sciences: The reformulated stepping-stone theory of heroin use as exemplar. *Journal of Personality and Social Psychology, 45,* 1289–1298.

Bell, R. Q. (1954). An experimental test of the accelerated longitudinal approach. *Child Development, 25,* 281–286.

Biddle, B. J., & Marlin, M. M. (1987). Causality, confirmation, credulity, and structural modeling. *Child Development, 58,* 4–17.

Bronfenbrenner, U. (1988). *Ecological systems theory.* Unpublished paper, Cornell University.

Bronfenbrenner, U., & Crouter, A. C. (1983). The evolution of environmental models in developmental research. In P. H. Mussen (Ed.), *Handbook of child psychology: Vol. I. History, theory, and methods* (W. Kessen, Volume editor) (pp. 357–414). New York: Wiley.

Carnegie Corporation (1988). *Summary of the third council meeting.* Held February 1–2, 1988, in Washington, D.C.

Elder, G. H., Jr., Caspi, A., & Downey, G. (1984a). Problem behavior and family relationships: Life course and intergenerational themes. In A. Sorenson, F. E. Weinert & L. Sherrod (Eds.), *Human development and the life course: Multidisciplinary perspectives* (pp. 293–340). Hillsdale, NJ: Erlbaum.

Elder, G. H., Jr., Liker, J. K., & Cross, C. E. (1984b). Parent-child behavior in the Great Depression: Life course and intergenerational influences. In P. B. Baltes & G. O. Brim (Eds.), *Life-span development and behavior, Vol. 6* (pp. 109–158). New York: Academic Press.

Galambos, N. L., & Silbereisen, R. K. (1987). Substance use in West German youth: A longitudinal study of adolescents' use of alcohol and tobacco. *Journal of Adolescent Research, 2,* 161–174.

Gold, M., & Petronio, J. P. (1980). Delinquent behavior in adolescence. In J. Adelson (Ed.), *Handbook of adolescent psychology.* New York: Wiley.

Gollob, H. F., & Reichardt, C. S. (1987). Taking account of time lags in causal models. *Child Development, 58,* 80–92.

Hertzog, C., & Nesselroade, J. R. (1987). Beyond autoregressive models: Some implications of the trait–state distinction for the structural modeling of developmental change. *Child Development, 58,* 93–109.

Jöreskog, K. G., & Sörbom, D. (1986). *Lisrel VI: Analysis of linear structural relationships by maximum likelihood, instrumental variables, and least square methods.* Mooresville, IN: Scientific Software.

Kandel, D. B., Mossel, P., & Kaestner, R. (1987). Drug use, the transition from school to work, and occupational achievement in the United States. *European Journal of Psychology of Education, 2,* 337–363 (Special Issue on *Adolescent Substance Use and Human Development,* R. K. Silbereisen & N. Galambos, Eds.)

Labouvie, E. W., & Nesselroade, J. R. (1988). *Representing change and process: Alternative structural models for longitudinal data.* Unpublished paper, Rutgers State University.

McArdle, J. J. (1988). Dynamic but structural equation modeling of repeated measures data. In J. R. Nesselroade & R. B. Cattell (Eds.), *Handbook of multivariate experimental psychology* (2nd ed.) (pp. 561–614). New York: Plenum.

McArdle, J., Anderson, E., & Aber, M. (1987). Convergence hypotheses modeled and tested with linear structural equations. In *Proceedings of the 1987 Public Health Conference on Records and Statistics* (pp. 347–352). Washington, DC: U.S. Department of Health and Human Services.

Nesselroade, J. R., & Baltes, P. B. (Eds.) (1979). *Longitudinal research in the study of behavior and development.* New York: Academic Press.

Petersen, A. C., & Crockett, L. J. (1985). Pubertal timing and grade effects on adjustment. *Journal of Youth and Adolescence, 14,* 191–206.

Rogosa, D. (1979). Causal models in longitudinal research: Rationale, formulation, and interpretation. In J. R. Nesselroade & P. B. Baltes (Eds.), *Longitudinal research in the study of behavior and development* (pp. 263–302). New York: Academic Press.

Rutter, M., & Garmezy, N. (1983). Developmental psychopathology. In E. M. Hetherington (Ed.), *Mussen's handbook of child psychology, Vol. 4. Socialization, personality and social development* (pp. 775–911). New York: Wiley.

Silbereisen, R. K., & Noack, P. (in press). On the constructive role of problem behavior in adolescence. In N. Bolger, A. Caspi, G. Downey, & M. Moorehouse (Eds.), *Person and context: Developmental processes.* Cambridge: Cambridge University Press.

Silbereisen, R. K., Petersen, A. C., Albrecht. H. T., & Kracke, B. (1988). *Maturational timing and the development of problem behavior: Longitudinal studies on adolescence.* Paper held at the XXIVth International Congress of Psychology, August 28–September 3, Sydney.

Silbereisen, R. K., & Reitzle, M. (in press). On the constructive role of problem behavior in adolescence: Further evidence on alcohol use. In L. P. Lipsitt & L. L. Mitnick (Eds.), *Self regulation, impulsivity, and risk-taking behavior: Causes and consequences.* Norwood, NJ: Ablex Publishing.

Silbereisen, R. K., & Walper, S. (1988 a). Person-process-context approaches. In M. Rutter (Ed.), *The power of longitudinal data: Studies of risk and protective factors for psychosocial disorders.* Cambridge, MA: Cambridge University Press.

Silbereisen, R. K., & Walper, S. (1988 b). The *role of social ties in coping with economic hardship.* Paper held at the Second Biennial Meetings of the Society for Research on Adolescence, March 25–27, Alexandria, VA.

Simmons, R. G., Blyth, D. A., & McKinney, K. L. (1983). The social and psychological effects of puberty on white females. In J. Brooks-Gunn & A. C. Petersen (Eds.), *Girls at puberty: Biological and psychosocial perspectives* (pp. 229–272). New York: Plenum.

Simmons, R. G., Burgeson, R., Carlton-Ford, S., & Blyth, D. A. (1987). The impact of cumulative change in early adolescence. *Child Development, 58,* 1220–1234.

Verdonik, F., & Sherrod, L. R. (1984). An *inventory of longitudinal research on childhood and adolescence.* New York: Social Science Research Council.

Walper, S., & Silbereisen, R. K. (1987 a). Individuelle und familiäre Konsequenzen ökonomischer Einbußen. *Zeitschrift für Entwicklungspsychologie und Pädagogische Psychologie, 19,* 1–21.

Walper, S., & Silbereisen, R. K. (1987 b). *Personal and contextual risk factors in coping with economic hardship.* Paper held at the IXth Biennial Meetings of the International Society for Research on Behavioral Development, July 12–16, Tokyo.

Child Psychiatric Research: On the Plurality of Approaches and Their Integration

Christopher Gillberg

Anyone who has ever been confronted with the narrow vision of enthusiastic researchers who have—or rather believe they have—just made a, or *the*, major breakthrough in their particular field will join me in sounding the bell of plurality. Anyone who has ever been subjected to the boring self-righteousness of the stubborn follower of one particular theory will feel the need to confront the demagogy that follows from such one-eyedness. Reference to the need for multiplicity—and often complexity—of methods and theories in child psychiatric research has been made countless time over the years and thus might sound trite, if not altogether obsolete. Nevertheless, it is important to keep repeating that many approaches—and not one—is the way forward in medicine generally and in child and adolescent psychiatry in particular. I remember when I was in training 20 years ago and my psychiatry professor made a plea for a multifactorial approach. I thought it sounded dull and opportunistic. But that plea, although not quite successful (in the sense that it has not yet been heeded by all and everybody) has not gone out of fashion. It has stood the test of time and remains to my mind the most important principle underlying any general concept of good child psychiatric research.

Some commonplace statements need to be made in this connection:

1. The child has a brain and a body. The mind and "soul" are complex phenomena, but in a sense they are ruled by the brain and limited or restricted by the body. This is not to say that the brain and body work independently of mind and soul. Indeed they do not. In point of fact, it has been proven beyond doubt that mind and body represent a reciprocal entity, the one influencing the other. What it does imply, however, is that good research in the field of child psychiatry cannot afford to ignore the brain and other biological factors. The future will test to what extent the brains and not only the bodies of boys are different from those of girls. In other words, sex differences should always be analyzed in psych-

iatric and—in particular—child and adolescent psychiatric research.

2. The child is a social creature and will always be influenced by social interactions in the widest sense of that word. Social measures must therefore be taken into account in child psychiatric research.

3. The child is a growing organism, which means that a developmental perspective needs to be applied, and that age and specificity must be considered.

4. The child experiences the social interactions in his/her mind differently at different ages. This psychological dimension is probably relatively less important in the newborn (although by no means necessarily unimportant), but becomes increasingly influential and differentiated as the child grows older. Intraindividual experiential factors will need a lot more systematic attention in the empiric studies of the future. So far, it has often been no more than anecdotal if anything.

The best child psychiatric research tries to incorporate all these four aspects in the design of a new study. However, rather often—for practical, financial, clinical, and other obvious reasons—the best cannot be attained. This paper is not intended as a pamphlet against all the studies that do not fit the ideal; we are dealing with realities, and we all know that usually the research we do is far from the ideal. Nevertheless, plurality of approaches need not necessarily be incorporated into one and the same study, although this would be the preferred route for future projects. Combinations of data from various studies may sometimes yield a comprehensive picture anyway. In the following, I will try to exemplify how a plurality of methods and theories can be applied in research projects in practice.

Plurality of Research Approaches

In child psychiatric research, a host of different avenues can be taken in order to get a little bit closer to the truth.

Epidemiological and in particular population-based research is and will remain the most important fundament in the delineation of syndromes, analysis of pathogenetic mechanisms, and follow-up of natural outcome. "One-step studies" with screening and examination of all possible cases are useful in research on rare problems. "Two-step studies" with screening of all possible cases and examination of a random sample are usually the best way of dealing with common syndromes.

Clinical studies of patient groups can be helpful in some respects, in particular if there is demographic data to show that the groups are typical or how they differ from the general norms of the unselected group. Clinical studies are useful when trying to draw attention to new aspects and can often provide important impetus for further research. Leo Kanner's first paper on autism (Kanner, 1943) provides a striking example of the terrible effects that clinical studies of highly biased groups can bring about. Not until the population-based studies of autism arrived on the scene in the 1970s and 1980s could we get rid of the dangerous notion of the cold mother which had been implanted by the clinical studies.

In this connection single-case studies should not be discarded as irrelevant, so long as their obvious limitations are acknowledged. They can still provide us with important clinical information, they can illustrate underlying principles, they are useful in defining diagnostic criteria, and they can indeed sometimes in themselves prove something in their own right. For instance, the appearance of an autistic syndrome in a previously healthy girl who at age 14 contacted herpes encephalitis *proves* that autistic symptoms can be caused by purely biological factors (Gillberg, 1986).

Experimental studies, including drug and other treatment studies, have their given place, but in order to get good generalizability of the results, a combination with an epidemiological approach is often best. Two recent pieces of top-class research illustrate the dilemma: Gerald Russell et al. (1987), in an ingenious study, showed that family therapy was an effective treatment method in anorexia nervosa. However, whether or not this conclusion is warranted for the whole population of anorexia nervosa cases remains an open question, since the experimental group was not a population-based one. Uta Frith and her group (Baron-Cohen et al., 1985) a few years ago presented fascinating evidence that the inability of conceiving other people as having minds might be a crucial dysfunction in autism. Whether or not this holds in autism generally is completely open to speculation because we have no way of knowing whether the groups of autistic children examined are representative or not.

Neurobiological, social, and psychological aspects need to be taken into account in all these fields of child psychiatric research. Even within these areas, there is a great need for plurality of approaches. Let me give you an example from one of my own fields. We have carried out comprehensive population-based studies of autism in Göteborg, Sweden. From the neurobiological point of view—which has been only one of several viewpoints—we were concerned that a too limited number of measures might leave us without the possibility of pin-pointing the crucial biological dysfunction in autism. Now, we are often warned not to use heavy artillery and shoot blindly into the woods. Using many measures might be taken by some to symbolize just that. But we thought—and eventually found—that there was no rational way of knowing just which particular measure would be better than all the others. We made use of CAT scans, auditory brainstem response examinations, EEGs, CSF analyses, blood and urine analyses, chromosomal cultures, ophthalmological, audiological, and otological examinations. Almost all the children were subjected to all or almost all the different examinations. This yielded data to show that virtually all the autistic children (compared with normal children) had signs of brain dysfunction, but no one method by itself detected more than 30–40% of the whole spectrum of problems. In using only CAT scans, for instance, Prior et al. (1984) concluded that high-functioning autistic kids have no signs of brain problems. Using all the methods just described, we found that 75% of the high-functioning autistic children have a major brain abnormality!

Plurality of Methods

Some of the possibly important neurobiological methods and measures that can and should be used in child psychiatric research are listed in Table 1.

There are, of course, a number of other neurobiological parameters, not the least in the clinical sphere. Thus, neurodevelopmental status, skin status, and general health status are usually important elements that should be included in all child psychiatric research. Ophthalmological, audiological, and otological examination have a place, too, much more so than currently accepted. In a study of teenage psychotic patients we found "trivial handicaps" such as refraction errors, hearing deficits, and a variety of relatively minor neuromuscular problems to be much more prevalent than in the general population

Table 1. Some neurobiological methods that may be valuable in child psychiatric research.

Method	Some examples of fields of proven or probable relevance
CAT scan	Autism
	Anorexia nervosa
	Mental retardation
NMR	Autism
	Mental retardation
(PET scan)*	Mental retardation
	Schizophrenia
SPECT	Autism
EEG	Behavior problems in epilepsy
	Situation-mediated changes in behavior
ABR (and other sensory-evoked potentials)	Autism
	Schizophrenia
Chromosomal cultures	Autism
	Speech-language disorders
	Learning disorders
CSF (protein, monoamines, endomorphins, amino acids)	Autism
	Atypical encephalitis
	Acute psychoses
Unine and blood analysis (e.g., monoamines)	Good potential in many fields
Reduced optimality scoring of pre-, peri-, and neonatal periods (Precht, 1980)	Clumsy children
	ADU
	Autism
	Teenage psychosis
	Mental retardation
	Tourette syndrome
Gene mapping	Autism

*difficult method requiring considerable technical expertise

(Hellgren et al., 1987). Such minor handicaps in combination with other factors, for instance, psychological trauma, might well predispose to the development even of severe psychopathology.

Which method(s) to use in a given study will depend on a number of things, such as hypothesis tested, availability, invasiveness of method and finding. The first thing the child psychiatrist has to do is to become acquainted with the range of possible methods and also the colleagues who use them. Collaboration on this level is the fundament without which no research in the field can be carried out.

I would like to say something here about the hopeless muddle we are presently in as regards terminology with respect to brain dysfunction. Over the years there have been many fruitless (and fruitful) discussions concerning the implication of "soft neurological signs" (e.g., Rutter, 1986). Statements to the effect that such signs do not indicate brain damage, though they might imply "genetic factors," are to me totally meaningless. Brain damage and hereditary factors may well—albeit on different routes—cause the same kind of neurochemical disturbance. Soft neurological signs, at least theoretically, could arise by any of the two routes and *must* be a sign of dysfunction or variation of brain activity.

In the field of social variables, countless methods, rating systems, scoring models, and questionnaires exist. It is beyond the scope of this paper to even try to give a comprehensive survey. Suffice it to say that at the start of any future research project in child psychiatry one will do well to consider carefully the type of social variables that are likely to shed some light on the problem studied. It is important always to remember that matching (e.g., a comparison group) for social variables usually precludes conclusions as to the contribution of these social factors. The need for a developmental approach in respect of studying social factors becomes evident if one compares ADHD and mania, for instance. In the former condition, the type of day care the child receives will be important, whereas in the latter, the school or work situation will be central instead.

Psychological methods range from tests of cognitive functioning to projective tests, self-rating questionnaires, and more or less structured clinical interviews. Many of the psychodynamically oriented tests used in clinical practice today have not been adequately tested for reliability and validity. This is sometimes taken as an excuse for discarding them altogether. I would be differently inclined and would rather advocate that, for example, tachistoscopic "Defence Mechanism Tests" (Kragh & Smith, 1970) and structural interviewing according to Kernberg (1984) be subjected to the same type of scientific scrutiny required in other fields. No doubt, we are in dire need of reliable and valid means of getting to know more about the experiential internal world of children and teenagers.

I turn now to look briefly at a few projects currently in progress in my own center.

Examples

Anorexia nervosa
(Plurality of General Approaches)

A major population-based study of anorexia nervosa (AN) is now being performed in Göteborg, Sweden. Using multiple screening measures (interviews with school nurse, school nurse examination of all pupils, questionnaires to all pupils, scrutiny of all growth charts, and a thorough register search) we believe that we have managed to trace all 15-year-olds with AN in Göteborg on December 15, 1985. These 20 cases, together with 20 more AN cases matched for sex, age, and a variety of other demographic variables with the population-based group, are followed up (as is indeed the whole population) and compared with 40 sex, age, and social class matched comparison cases on a variety of biological, social, and psychological variables. All 80 youngsters are subjected to a neurobiological work-up including detailed physical examination, EEG, chromosomal culture, hormone analyses, and other specific blood and urine tests, such as zink. The social variables studied are too numerous to even begin to list them in this context. Psychologically, we rely on the clinical psychiatric interview with each teenager and the mother (together some 2 hours), the EAT, the Birleson depression inventory (Birleson, 1981), the Eysenck inventory (Eysenck & Eysenck, 1964), and the modified FACES covering aspects of family structure suggested by Olsson and Cederbladh (unpublished manuscript, 1986). All in all, we hope that this will provide us with a broad basis for follow-up and for some pathogenetic speculation. Using only one approach, e.g., a psychological, would have meant that we would be stuck in a situation in which the possible influence of biological and social factors could not be reasonably assessed at all. Preliminary data from this study indicates that AN in Sweden has its peak age of onset at 14 years, affects more than 1% of all teenage girls and 0.1% of all boys, that social class is no different than in the general population, that many are clinically depressed, that private schools have a much higher rate of AN, that chromosomes (including sex-chromatin) are normal, and that the families often—though by no means always—regard themselves as "among the happiest in the world" (Råstam et al., 1988; Råstam, personal communication, 1988).

DAMP
(Plurality of Psychological Approaches)

In our 10-year follow-up of population-based groups of originally 6-year-old children with Deficits in Attention, Motor control and Perception (DAMP) and their comparison groups (e.g., Gillberg, I.C. 1987), we are using a variety of psychological methods in order to tap intrapsychic and personality problems that we expect to be very frequent in the DAMP group. We use a DSM-III-R interview designed by Loranger et al. (1986) and modified for Swedish teenagers by ourselves (Bågenholm et al., 1987) in order to elicit enough data to be able to make a DSM-III-R diagnosis according to axis I and II. The teenagers complete a Swedish version of the MCMI (Millon, 1983), which yields subscores for classification of personality disorders. A "blinded" psychiatrist makes a one-hour video-taped interview according to Kernberg and then administers a tachistoscopic *Defence Mechanism Test* (DMT). The different methods are then comprehensively evaluated and a global diagnosis made by yet an independent psychiatrist. Employing all these different measures, they can also be used to validate each other. For example, will the structural interview (which is entirely focused on the *interaction* between the proband and the interviewer) yield enough information to warrant a diagnosis of borderline personality disorder in all cases thus diagnosed on the basis of the highly structured DSM-III-R interview (which is almost entirely symptom-oriented)?

Teenage Psychosis/Borderline Conditions
(Plurality of Screening Methods)

In order to ascertain a population-based group of all cases of operationally defined psychosis and borderline personality disorder (DSM-III-R) among 16- and 17-year-olds in Göteborg at a chosen census date, we are using a variety of screening devices. The school nurse interviews each teacher, who in turn completes the Swedish versions of the *Newcastle Adolescent Behaviour Scale* designed by Place et al. (1987) for each teenager who is not immediately and definitely regarded as without moderate or major emotional or behavioral problems. The registers of child and adolescent psychiatric as well as adult psychiatric out- and inpatient clinics are searched, and all the doctors in these clinics personally interviewed in accordance with a structured manual containing, among others, the questions suggested by Khouri et al. (1980) for the screening of borderline and psychotic conditions. By using a broad approach like this, we feel confident that not many true cases will be lost by the identification procedure. Using only one of the four methods might well prove to be either adequate or totally inadequate. Time will tell!

Table 2. Example: Autism (integration of approaches). Findings in a case of an 8-year-old boy with autism and mild mental retardation.

Method	Possible finding
Clinical psychosocial interview data	No friends
	Parents disagree regarding child's degree of handicap
	Sibling depressed
Frith "doll test" (Baron-Cohen et al., 1985)	Failure
WISC	Extreme deficits in picture arrangements and word comprehension
Physical state including skin at age 8 years	Normal
CSF	High HVA:HMPG quotient
EEG	Subcortical epileptogenic activity
ABR	Prolonged brainstem transmission time
NMR	Widening of fourth ventricle
CAT scan	Periventricular calcification
Chromosomal culture	Doubtful, chromosome 9 abnormality detectable in near future?
RFLP (family)	Linkage "chromosome 9 probe"
Follow-up 5 years later	Adenoma sebaceum

Autism
(Plurality of Biological Methods)

I have already indicated why it is sometimes necessary to include a wide variety of neurobiological examinations in the study of a particular disorder. In the—to my mind—misguided intention to find *one* clue to the riddle of autism, far too many researchers set out to study autistic children using this or that "specific" method. Many came out of such undertakings with a disappointed shrug of the shoulders: Nothing specific turned up. We and others have shown that by using a wide range of neurobiological assessment methods, autism has become less puzzling. Just as with mental retardation, it is now clear that autism is caused by a variety of different agents, ranging from

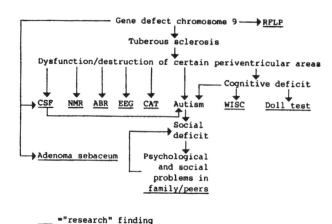

Figure 1. Integration of findings from Table 2.

___ ▪"research" finding

PKU and tuberous sclerosis to the fragile-X-syndrome and herpes encephalitis (Gillberg, 1988). This current state of the art would never have been achieved had we not relied on a plurality of neurobiological approaches. Autism provides a good example of how, in the early stages of the history of a disorder, a plurality of approaches rather than much revered specific hypothesis testing is called for.

Table 2 and Figure 1 exemplify how multilevel research methods and data can be applied and integrated in a case of autism gradually discovered to be caused by tuberous sclerosis and in itself causing distress, psychological and social problems. The model is applied to a single case for reasons of simplicity and clarity, but is, of course, applicable in research on child psychiatric populations.

Plurality of Theories

Are theories really necessary in child psychiatric research? Yes, of course, they are, at least as a framework for ordering ideas and empirical data. But they should never be an end in themselves and certainly must incorporate empirical findings in the constant reformulation of new, or rather redefined, theories. We need biological theories and social theories and psychological theories and a whole host of "subtheories" within these fields. It sounds like stating the obvious, but one is constantly reminded of the necessity—in clinical practice and research—of always considering child psychiatric problems from more than one angle.

Future Trends

Who knows what the future holds? How can the different theories and plurality of methods be integrated? In this day and age, on the threshold of the era of the new genetics, there is no telling where we may stand even as soon as the year 2000. But let me give you an example of how psychological and biological research have long developed in a parallel fashion in the field of autism and how now, at last, the two lines seem to be converging. The psychological studies provide tentative evidence for a rather specific psychological deficit in autism, viz. that of not being able to conceive of other people's perspectives or even that they have a separate mind. The biological studies are gradually closing in on the brain areas likely to be dysfunctional in autism. It is our hope now that findings from psychologists will refine the methods and narrow the search for the neurobiological substrate and vice versa. In other fields, too, I expect similar fertilizing interaction.

References

American Psychiatric Association (1987). *DSM-III-R. Diagnostic and Statistical Manual of Mental Disorders* (3rd, rev. ed.). Washington, DC: Author.

Baron-Cohen, S., Leslie, A. M., & Frith, U. (1985). Does the autistic child have a "theory of mind"? *Cognition, 21,* 37–46.

Birleson, P. (1981). The validity of depressive disorder in childhood and the development of a self-rating scale: A research report. *Journal of Child Psychology and Psychiatry, 22,* 73–88.

Eysenck, H. J., & Eysenck, S. S. G. (1964). *Manual of the Eysenck Personality Inventory.* London: University of London Press.

Gillberg, C. (1986). Brief report: Onset at age 14 of typical autistic syndrome. A case report of a girl with herpes simplex encephalitis. *Journal of Autism and Developmental Disorders, 16,* 369–375.

Gillberg, C. (1988). The neurobiology of infantile autism. *Journal of Child Psychology and Psychiatry, 29,* 257–266.

Gillberg, I. C. (1987). *Deficits in attention, motor control and perception: Follow-up from pre-school to the early teens.* Thesis, Uppsala University.

Hellgren, L., Gillberg, C., & Enerskog, I. (1987). Antecedents of teenage psychoses. A population-based study of school health problems in children who develop psychosis in teenage. *Journal of the American Academy of Child Psychiatry, 26,* 351–355.

Kanner, L. (1943). *Childhood psychosis. Initial studies and new insights.* Washington, DC: Winston.

Kernberg, O. (1984). *Severe personality disorders. Psychotherapeutic strategies.* New Haven/London: Yale University Press.

Khouri, P. J., Haier, R. J., Rieder, R. O., & Rosenthal, D. (1980). A symptom schedule for the diagnosis of borderline schizophrenia. A first report. *British Journal of Psychiatry, 137,* 140–147.

Kragh, U., & Smith, G. (Eds.) (1970). *Percept-genetic analysis.* Lund: Gleerup.

Loranger, A. W., Susman, V. L., Oldham, J. M., & Russakoff, L. M. (1986). *Personality Disorder Examination (PDE): A structured interview for DSM-III-R personality disorders. Adolescent version.* The New York Hospital–Cornell Medical Center, White Plains, NY. Swedish version: Bågenholm, A., Gillberg, C., Hellgren, L., & Ivarson, T. (1987).

Millon, T. (1983). *Millon Clinical Multiaxial Inventory Manual* (3rd. ed.).

Place, M., Kolvin, I., & Morton, S. M. (1987). Newcastle Adolescent Behaviour Screening Questionnaire. *British Journal of Psychiatry, 151,* 45–51.

Prechtl, H. F. R. (1980). The optimality concepts. *Early Human Development, 4,* 201–205.

Prior, M. R., Tress, B., Hoffman, W. L., & Boldt, D. (1984). Computer tomographic study of children with classic autism. *Archives of Neurology, 41,* 482–484.

Råstam, M., Gillberg, C., & Gahrton, M. (1989). Anorexia nervosa in a Swedish urban region. A population-based study. *British Journal of Psychiatry.* Accepted for publication.

Russell, G. F. M., Szmukler, G. I., Dare, C., & Eisler, I. (1987). An evaluation of family therapy in anorexia nervosa and bulimia nervosa. *Archives of General Psychiatry, 44,* 1047–1056.

Rutter, M. (1986). Looking 30 years ahead. *Journal of Child Psychology and Psychiatry, 27,* 803–840.

SECTION II:

THE MATURING INDIVIDUAL FACING PATHOGENIC INFLUENCES

Externalizing Disorders: Priorities for Future Research

Eric Taylor

Risk Factors for Disruptive Behavior

Most children referred for psychiatric help are sent not because of their personal suffering, but because of their disruptiveness toward others. Many studies have indicated differences between them and children showing overt emotional distress. Statistically, the defiant, noncompliant, antisocial, and aggressive behavior problems tend to cluster together and to segregate from anxiety, misery, and somatizing symptoms. Many of the associations considered below, such as a high male-to-female ratio, a strong link to signs of adversity in family life, and a strong tendency to persist over time characterize disruptive children but not the emotionally upset.

The words "externalizing" and "internalizing" are often used to refer to these two major subtypes of dysfunction. They are best used only to convey the overt behavior patterns. Their use, however, can also lead to a tacit acceptance of an unproven theory: that disruptive behavior results from acting out the same types of inner conflict that cause emotional upset. For that reason, I generally use "disruptive" and not "externalized" below, to mean the broad type of disturbance that includes aggressive, hyperactive patterns of behavior.

The attempt to understand and help children who are at odds with the expectations of society now has a long and honorable history. Child psychiatry had its very beginnings in the effort to treat children referred by the courts. Epidemiological, longitudinal, clinical, and therapeutic trial techniques have all been used with profit. There is now a rich knowledge about the many associations of disruptive behavior and a useful framework of knowledge for beginning to understand its evolution over time. There are also many reviews of the scientific work (e.g., Garmezy & Rutter, 1983), so I can survey previous work with some brevity and with reference chiefly to reviews rather than primary sources. I indicate mostly where puzzles remain rather than attempting a comprehensive consensus of findings.

The main research issues for the immediate future seem to me to be those that could advance knowledge beyond the description of associations to an understanding of how risk factors work. Many factors are considered to influence an antisocial development. But which of them are independent agents and which are simply markers to more fundamental risk factors? Do all factors operate by contributing to a single outcome? Or is there a typology of disruptive disorders, with differentiated types of risk? There is a strong continuity of antisociality through childhood and adolescence, even though children change enormously over the same years. What explains the continuity? Long-term change is hard to achieve, even when programs of intervention are effective in the short term. What then should be the goals of treatment? The paradox of the subject area is the combination of extensive knowledge of the determinants of disorder with the relatively small impact of most evaluated treatments on individuals. This conflict should be the spur to developing less orthodox therapy, and social interventions—and to understanding the mediators of continuity more deeply.

Reviewing risks and their modification is at once complicated by the fragmentation of the literature. Hyperactivity (or ADDH) has generated one volume of research; delinquency another; aggression and conduct disorders a third and fourth; substance abuse another volume again. Yet, as I argue, the people studied by these traditions are so similar that it is highly artificial to consider them in separate chapters of a textbook or in unconnected research projects. Most hyperactive children are conduct-disordered, most conduct-disordered hyperactive (Taylor, 1988 a). The hyperactive are at high risk for later substance abuse and delinquency (Gittelman et al., 1985; Satterfield et al., 1982). Indeed, in a recent U.S.-U.K. diagnostic study of DSM-III and ICD 9 diagnoses applied to disruptive boys, there was very little agreement between clinicians on which of the boys should be categorized as hyperactive, which as conduct disordered, and which as both (Prendergast et al., 1988). When both types of problem are present, U.K. clinicians tend to see the disorder as one of conduct, U.S. clinicians as one of activity control. Accordingly, recent reviewers have seen an immediate issue of research as one of attempting a valid subtyping of the heterogeneous disorders that present with disruptive conduct (e.g., Rutter, 1988; Werry et al., 1987; Taylor, 1988 a).

Table 1 sets out some of the known associates of disruptive conduct in terms of qualities of the child that are conventionally used in descriptions of psychopathology, other qualities of the child, and aspects of his or her social environment. The list is not comprehensive and omits some interesting findings from case-control studies (e.g., of EEG changes) whose specificity is unclear. It also omits considerations of outcome and longitudinal course, since these have been dealt with in the previous chapter.

Table 1. Some associations of disruptive conduct in children.

I. Child psychopathology	II. Other qualities of child	III. Social and family background
restless, inattentive behavior	male gender	urban environment
impulsiveness	reading disability	school atmosphere
poor peer relationship	low scores on IQ and neuropsychological tests	antisocial relatives
affective disturbance		size of sibship
delinquency,	muscularity	marital discord
substance abuse		between parents
	tissue lead	*parental:*
	plasma testosterone	rejection
	catecholamine metabolism altered	punitiveness
	minor neurological abnormalities	hostility
	diminished psycho- physiological respon- siveness	permissiveness
	difficult temperament	
	social understanding altered	coerciveness
	rare: brain damage, chromosome change	

Associated Risk Factors: Psychopathology

Children referred for specialist help because of disruptive, aggressive, hyperactive, or otherwise troublesome behavior very often show other problems as well. In part this is because the other problems have contributed to the referral; but epidemiological studies have also illustrated the degree of overlap (Taylor, 1988 b). Some of the overlap is, of course, a matter of definition. It is not surprising if disruptive children find themselves in trouble with the law. But it is not inevitable, and a high proportion of the ordinary population of boys in cities are delinquent in the broad sense of receiving a conviction for a minor offence.

The frequency of comorbidity is important. It means, for example, that intervention services have to be broadly based and draw upon a range of approaches and professional disciplines. It also limits the value of simple case-control designs— especially of those where cases are referred and controls are not. Population-based studies are likely to play an increasingly dominant role in understanding the externalizing disorders.

Since so many problems can be present, it is often hard to know which of them is the key to a dependent variable that is being studied. Are neuropsychological impairments, for example, associated with antisociality, aggression, hyperactivity, poor peer relationships, or a subgroup of conduct-disordered children who will become adult psychopaths? Studies could be cited in support of all these views, and of course it is conceivable that all of them will prove to be related in different ways to brain dysfunction. However, the coexistence of the different problems in the same children means that we have all too little information about the discriminative prediction of different types of problem. It would be wrong to conclude from these studies that all the problems have the same associations and are part of a unitary disorder. This could still be true, but the only reasonable conclusion in current evidence is that we do not know.

One research approach to this confused situation is a multivariate strategy, in which (for example) hyperactivity and defiance have been shown to have differential associations with impairment of psychological test performance when the other is allowed for (Loney et al., 1978). Another approach is the definition of pure, homogeneous groups who show (for example) only hyperactivity or only conduct disorder without the other problem. From one such study the same conclusion about the independence of hyperactivity and conduct disorder has been drawn (Taylor, 1988 b). Both these strategies will be needed in the future. However, the adoption of either strategy means that the investigators already have a good idea of the key variables to use in the classification. The distinction between hyperactivity and conduct disorder does seem to be important (albeit not all studies have found it; vide Werry et al., 1987). However, there are many other possible ways of slicing the cake. This requires a systematic approach to understanding the relationships of clinical variables and the clustering of cases.

Subtyping according to types of offensive behavior seems to have relatively little value. There is a possible distinction between aggression (as seen at home) and uncomplicated stealing (outside home). But it is not clear whether differences—in family background and outcome—arise from that or from the distinction acting as a marker for other more fundamental differences. Similarly, hyperactivity may falsely appear to have specific associations because its presence is also a marker to increased severity of conduct disorder (Taylor, 1988 b). Similar problems arise for the suggested subdivisions of unsocialized vs socialized; aggressive vs nonaggressive; stress-related vs non-stress-related; or for those based on motivational or personality variables (Garmezy & Rutter, 1983). No subdivision has fared very well against the criterion of predicting longitudinal course: Number of problems seems a better guide than type. However, it is quite possible that the severity of conduct disorder is the main determinant of outcome, although there are several distinguishable routes into conduct disorder, with etiological factors operating in several ways. If so, subtyping is deeply relevant to etiology and early prevention, but largely irrelevant to course, treatment, and tertiary prevention.

Problems and Approaches for the Subtyping of Disorders

There are several obstacles to a good classification. The first of these is the ambiguity that has crept into some descriptive terms such as "impulsiveness" and "attention deficit" (Taylor, 1986). Both can refer to behavioral or cognitive constructs, or to supposed underlying disorders. Clinicians may think they know what they mean; in practice, they do not all mean the same thing (Prendergast et al., 1988). This situation seems to cry out for an ethological approach using direct observation and carefully described behavioral categories. The beginnings of this process have indicated some agreement between what is carefully observed and what is rated by a clinician (Dienske et al., 1985; Luk et al., 1987). The future of this research should not be to judge observation against clinicians' ratings, but to refine clinicians' ratings to agree with observation. It will also allow for more detailed and subtle analysis of behaviors such as coercion, protest, distractibility, and orienting of attention.

Other tools of assessment also need development. Rating scales are now quite good, comprehensive tools for the screening of populations, the monitoring of treatment, and for some kinds of group comparisons. But they include several sources of error and are insufficient for individual diagnosis. Detailed, behavioral interview accounts by people who know the child well as well as direct observational techniques are likely to represent the way forward. They will need to be standardized for different ages, IQ levels, and gender. They will be costly in time and thus will not replace the rating scale approach; but they will allow for clearer specification of the targets for treatment and education. The analysis of peer relationships will need not only a development of observational measures, but also of children's self-reports to give measures of their understanding of themselves and other people.

Another obstacle to a good classification is the uncertainty over what sort of dimensions, or categories, should be recognized. As one example, I think that there is now considerable evidence that a subgroup of inattentive and restless children should be identified as a hyperkinetic disorder; but the size of the subgroup and the clinical qualities that should define it are still matters of debate (Rutter, 1988). The broad category of ADDH in DSM-III is not satisfactory, and should not be retained (Rutter, 1988; Taylor, 1988 a). However, the revision of "ADDH" into "ADHD" in DSM-III-R does not seem to make matters much better. The criteria proposed for "hyperkinetic disorder" in ICD 10 seem more useful and have received some support by the ability of a restricted definition of hyperkinesis to predict neuropsychological impairment, language delays, clumsiness, and early onset in a recent epidemiological study (Taylor, 1988 b), and to predict similar impairments and a marked response to stimulant medication in a clinical study (Taylor et al., 1986).

As another example, there is considerable evidence that there are biological causes for at least a subgroup of disruptive children (especially those with hyperkinetic disorder). Nevertheless, the idea of a minimal brain dysfunction syndrome is much too grand, does not correspond with the lack of association between its supposed components (Schmidt et al., 1987), and muddles supposed etiology with clinical aspects in an unproductive fashion that does not square with experimental work. As yet another instance, many clinicians would agree on the presence of depressive symptoms in some disruptive children, and depression has appeared as the main feature of one subgroup of disruptive children in a cluster analytic study (Taylor et al., 1986). There is, however a dearth of evidence on what the criteria should be for the identification of such a group.

Future research should plan clustering studies based on representative groups and etiological studies of homogeneous subgroups, so that the most sharply predictive subtyping can survive at the expense of the others.

A linked problem for classification is the uncertainty about just what level of symptomatology needs to exist before a subject can be classified as a "case." This problem is more severe since it turns out that problems such as defiant conduct and attention deficit are continuously distributed as dimensions in the population, so that no obvious cut-off point exists (Taylor, 1988 b). It will therefore be necessary to assess the predictive value of different grades of severity in different populations for overall social adjustment.

A fourth obstacle to a successful nosology is the problem of comorbidity between types of dysfunction, mentioned above. Preliminary evidence and clinical experience seem to argue that mixtures of problems are the rule, but it is necessary to test this idea and to enquire about the meaning and implications of overlap. Indeed, the meaning of different kinds of overlap may well be rather different, so that the issues will be in rather different form for the overlaps between (for example) defiant conduct on the one hand, and hyperactivity, attention deficit, depression, learning disorders, and multiple tics on the other.

Next, there is still considerable uncertainty about the relationships between several of the recognized symptom patterns in this area. To take just the central example of attention disturbance, what is the relationship of "attention deficit disorder with hyperactivity" (ADD-H) to the severe hyperkinetic syndrome encountered in some intellectually retarded children? What is the relationship between attention deficit disorder and the probable deficiency of attention in those at high risk for schizophrenia? Is attention deficit alone (i.e., without hyperactivity or conduct disorder) the same problem as when it occurs in combination? This kind of question—which is crucial for considering who should be given prevention or treatment—requires the systematic comparison of differently defined groups and longitudinal studies.

Sixth, there is still some uncertainty concerning the meaning of changes of symptom picture with time. If a child with clear hyperactivity develops into an older child with conduct disorder and a young adult with immature personality disorder, how are these concepts related? Are the earlier conditions embryonic forms of the later? Or age-appropriate manifestations of the same thing? Or diffuse risk factors whose outcome is determined by later events? Those questions require the prospective application of repeated measures to a longitudinally studied group. Since this kind of work is notoriously expensive, it would be prudent to develop clarity of case-defining schemes before embarking upon the full program.

The research envisaged by this section is likely to help in understanding the conceptual nature of a useful nosology. Should it be based on mutually exclusive categories, or upon hierarchies of categories? More meaningfully, for what different purposes are these different styles of classification best fitted? On what grounds should one differentiate between them?

Risk Factors in Children and Their Backgrounds

The theme of subtyping, considered above, is close to that of the specificity or diffuseness of risk factors. Many of the associated factors illustrated in the second and third columns of Table 1 need to be mapped against subtypes of disorder and against each other.

One of the clearest examples of this process has been the study of the relationship between the exposure to lead and the presence of behavior disturbance. There has been a general agreement that high tissue lead levels are weakly correlated with disruptive behavior and psychological test impairment. It has also been generally recognized that high lead levels are a marker to social disadvantage as well as being potentially harmful in themselves. The causative pathway is therefore obscure.

This is a common situation for the factors known to be associated with conduct problems. The unusual aspect of the lead work is that its political (rather than medical) importance has attracted enough funding to allow for the types of study that will be important. Several groups of investigators have reported multiple regression analyses, in which the association between lead and behavior is examined after allowing for the effects of adverse social circumstances (see Silva et al., 1988, as a recent example). It is not my purpose here to review the results; most seem to find that the association is attenuated but still statistically significant after the statistical controls have been made. Rather, I wish to highlight the importance of the research strategy and also its limitations.

Some of the disagreement comes because of technical differences. Thus, the more factors that are controlled for, the greater becomes the risk of overcorrection in the multiple regression. Obviously, too, the choice of factors to be controlled for may on the one hand miss the key environmental circumstances or, on the other hand, remove the influence of lead itself. Some of the disagreement comes because the effect size is small, and often on the very boundary of statistical significance with the sample sizes taken. It would be a better strategy to focus attention on factors of large effect first.

However, even when technical considerations are solved, there are still problems of interpretation. Children's behavior may itself increase their exposure to lead (as may be implied by the higher levels of blood lead in boys than in girls). The causal relationship may therefore run from behavior to the supposed risk factor. It is therefore desirable to seek groups of children in whom exposure to lead is determined by factors obviously *not* the consequence of their behavior (e.g., their geographical proximity to a newly started industrial source of pollution), and (again) to use a longitudinal strategy.

It is, in short, an arduous and expensive business to determine the details of pathogenesis even of a single well-defined factor; yet the details of pathogenesis are crucial for decisions about prevention and treatment. This general lesson can be drawn from many of the associated factors of Table 1.

Consider, for example, the clustering of antisocial relatives in the families of disruptive children. The finding is clear, both for those regarded as showing conduct disorder and for those diagnosed as having hyperactivity or ADDH (Taylor, 1986). The reasons for the association are not clear.

Is there a genetic link? The Scandinavian adoptive study described by Bohman and Sigvardsson (1980) and reanalyzed by Bohman et al. (1982) suggested that there was indeed a genetic inheritance of something related to conduct disorder (though separate from alcoholism). On the other hand, an adoptive study of the offspring of psychiatrically disturbed or normal parents suggested a genetically inherited link between childhood hyperactivity and the whole spectrum of mental illness in their parents (Cunningham et al., 1975). There have been several studies of relatives of hyperactive children, but the results are not in any way conclusive. I will not review them here in detail: to do so would be to repeat the major methodological weaknesses noted by the authors and frequently emphasized since by reviewers. Neither —again, because of methodological weaknesses—will I put any stress on the finding from the previously cited epidemiological study in London, namely, that antisocial relatives clustered with non-hyperactive but conduct-disordered probands, not with hyperkinetic probands—though it does seem possible that hyperkinetic disorder does not tend to affect several children in the same family, unlike delinquency (Taylor, 1988 b). Rather, I wish to emphasize the gap in the literature. The techniques are now in place for genetic studies using family pedigree, twin and adoption designs, and the methods of molecular genetics. They have considerable promise for clarifying what is inherited, the subtyping of disorders, and whether the familial association is for a temperamental attribute (e.g., of activity or "difficulty") or for a psychiatric syndrome. They should be an early priority in research.

It is, however, unlikely that genetic inheritance accounts for the whole of the association with adverse aspects of family life. In clinical studies, defiant conduct is linked quite closely to negative expressed emotion, inconsistency between parents, and impaired levels of parental coping (Taylor et al., 1986). In the general population, the same factors are found in association both with hyperkinetic disorder and non-hyperactive conduct disorder (Taylor, 1988 b). These are factors operating for the individual child, rather than across the entire family, and may well represent family reactions to behavioral deviation rather than the initiating cause. Once established, however, they probably form part of the family adversities and maladaptive patterns of parent-child interaction that are known to predict poor outcome for hyperactive children (Weiss & Hechtman, 1986). Perhaps they represent part of the way that children's constitutions shape their environments (Scarr & McCartney, 1985). Improved measures of family function should therefore be applied primarily to the longitudinal issue of how qualities of children interact with the way they are treated to determine outcome.

For this purpose, it will be desirable to establish and follow-up the relatively rare groups of children who have good family function in spite of their disruptiveness, and vice versa, as well as the usual groups of children who show problems in both domains or in neither. Intervention studies (see below) also offer the chance of modifying family factors, and effective interventions would be a helpful way of determining what is causative.

Schachar et al. (1987) have described a lessening of negative expressed emotion by parents when disruptive children were successfully treated with methylphenidate. The ability of intervention at one level to alter processes at another both suggests how effective treatments might be developed and gives an approach to studying process.

Many other associations of hyperactivity, aggression, defiance and antisocial conduct can now generate programs of research to clarify the mediating processes:

— The higher prevalence in males is a highly robust finding: Comparisons of affected males with affected females could suggest why. If the reasons stem from the different ways in which boys and girls are treated, they would be a useful indication of which features in the psychological environment should be targets for modification.

— Differences between neighborhoods in the prevalence of behavior problems are known and strong: Urban-rural differences are known for many types of psychiatric pathology (Quinton, 1988), but they seem to be especially strong for disorders involving hyperactive behavior (Boyle et al., 1987). They are presumably generated by coexisting disadvantage rather than the urban environment per se: a disadvantaged rural population in mainland China had higher rates of ADDH than did an urban population (Shen et al., 1985). One set of major factors operating is probably those causing the family problems already mentioned (Quinton, 1988), but they may also work through variations in the effectiveness of schools.

— Impairments of neuropsychological function are linked particularly to the inattentive component of disorder, and especially to the restricted definition of hyperkinetic disorder.

This conclusion, and the validation of a reliable case-finding scheme, opens up several lines of studying the etiology of the hyperkinetic subgroup. Brain-imaging studies and quantitative EEG analyses are powerful tools that can now be deployed upon a promising group of cases.

The effect of stimulant medication upon the disorder is one clue, and investigations of neurotransmitter metabolism are correspondingly relevant. Such studies have, of course, begun to be reported about ADDH; but they are both scanty and contradictory in their findings (see Oades, 1987, for a review). Even the studies that have been done are of limited relevance to our knowledge about a restricted hyperkinetic disorder. Greater clarity of findings could be expected from the study of a more biologically determined group.

The association with a rather global pattern of cognitive impairment suggests a different line of investigation from the studies of information processing that now make up the central tradition of experimental psychological research into ADDH. The behaviors involved in attending should also become a subject for experimental analysis. This will require closer descriptions of behaviors such as orientation, search, scanning, and preferences, their developmental course, the factors that determine them, and how they relate to difficulties in learning.

The more usually adopted experimental techniques, of studying information processing, have not yet suggested a specific structural deficiency in the processing of information or in the processes of attention (Douglas, 1983). Nevertheless, such research still has some merit, especially in exploring processes linked to motivation and inhibition of impulsive responding. Some experimental ingenuity will be needed, to devise variations in test procedure that can alter bad test performance to good and even lead to a superior performance by those in "pathological" groups.

Other research at the level of individual pathology may very usefully focus upon the information processing that underlies social competence and incompetence with other children. A current example comes from the work of Dodge et al. (1987), who have conceived of social behavior as a function of children's processing social environmental cues through encoding, mental representation, accessing potential responses, selecting a good response and enacting it. They set competent and incompetent children to watch videotapes of children interacting and, separately, to enact a similar situation. Processing skill predicted actual performance, and better performance was associated with natural popularity. Processing about a peer group entry situation did not predict aggression; but processing about a situation involving provocation was indeed associated with more aggression. The enhancement of social processing may come to join the armamentarium of therapeutic interventions. This is difficult research, and the determinants of performance will need to be specified. The situation-specificity of much disruptive behavior should be a caution against over-rapid acceptance of any general explanation based on individual pathology. One of the goals of research is to clarify the situational as well as the personal determinants of behavior.

Summary

In this chapter I have touched on the need for a wide range of studies. They have included the improvement of the means of assessment, their application to representative series of cases, and the use of the techniques of numerical taxonomy; the etiological study of homogeneous subtypes of disorder; the use of multivariate and longitudinal designs for short-term outcome studies; an expansion of genetic work and of work on intra-familial process; epidemiological comparisons of high- and low-prevalence populations; developmental psychological approaches to children's understanding of relationships and use of their knowledge; and studies of those children whose disruptive behavior is specific to a situation, with particular reference to the situational determinants.

This is, of course, a formidable shopping list. It would be even longer had I included the outcome and intervention studies that are to be discussed in other chapters. The length of the list, however, reflects the excitement and interest of the subject area. Concepts and methods have advanced to the point where most of the studies could be usefully mounted at once, or with only relatively brief preparation and refinement of measures and subject groups.

It will, nevertheless, be important that these studies be done within a collaborative framework of subject description so that one investigation is readily understandable by other investigators. This has not always been the case. Researchers should be enabled to work across centers and adopt compatible tools of measurement. Furthermore, the research envisaged is nearly all multidisciplinary. This seems to imply that funding agencies should consider the support of a few groups of investigators who can bring continuity to the research scene. This should not, of course, totally replace the reactive style of funding in which investigator-generated projects are judged competitively. Nevertheless, the field is now so rich in one-off projects that the virtues of a programmatic approach have become evident.

References

Bohman, M., & Sigvardsson, S. (1980). A prospective longitudinal study of children registered for adoption. *Acta Psychiatrica Scandinavica, 61,* 339–355.

Bohman, M., Cloninger, C. R., Sigvardsson, S., & von Knorring, A.-L. (1982). Predisposition to petty criminality in Swedish adoptees : I. Genetic and environmental heterogeneity. *Archives of General Psychiatry, 29,* 1233–1241.

Boyle, M. H., Offord, D. R. et al. (1987). Ontario Child Health Study : I. Methodology and II. Six-month prevalence of disorder and rates of service utilisation. *Archives of General Psychiatry, 44,* 826–836.

Cunningham, L., Cadoret, R., Loftus, R., & Edwards, J. E. (1975). Studies of adoptees from psychiatrically disturbed biological parents. *British Journal of Psychiatry, 126,* 534–539.

Dienske, H., de Jonge, G., & Sanders-Woudstra, J. A. R. (1985). Quantitative criteria for attention and activity in child psychiatric patients. *Journal of Child Psychology and Psychiatry, 26,* 895–916.

Dodge, K. A., Pettit, G. S., & Braun, M. M. (1987). Social competence in children. *Monographs of the Society for Research in Child Development, 51,* No. 2.

Douglas, V. (1983). Attentional and cognitive problems. In M. Rutter (Ed.), *Developmental neuropsychiatry.* New York: Guilford Press.

Garmezy, N., & Rutter, M. (1983). *Stress, coping, and development in children.* San Francisco: McGraw-Hill.

Gittelman, R., Mannuzza, S., Sheriker, R., & Bonagura, N. (1985). Hyperactive boys almost grown up: I. Psychiatric status. *Archives of General Psychiatry, 42,* 937–947.

Loney, J., Langhorne, J., & Paternite, C. (1978). An empirical basis for subgrouping the hyperkinetic/minimal brain dysfunction syndrome. *Journal of Abnormal Psychology, 87,* 431–441.

Luk, S.-L., Thorley, G., & Taylor, E. (1987). Gross overactivity: A study by direct observation. *Journal of Psychopathology and Behavioral Assessment, 9*(2), 173–182.

Oades, R.D. (1987). Attention deficit disorder with hyperactivity (ADDH): The contribution of catecholaminergic activity. *Progress in Neurobiology, 29,* 365–391.

Predergast, M., Taylor, E. A., Rapoport, J. L., Bartteo, J., Donnelly, M., Zametkin, A., Ahearn, M. B., Dunn, G., & Wieselberg, H. M. (1988). The diagnosis of childhood hyperactivity: A U.S.–U.K. cross-national study of DSM-III and ICD 9. *Journal of Child Psychology and Psychiatry, 29,* 289–300.

Quinton, D. (1988). Annotation: Urbanism and child mental health. *Journal of Child Psychology and Psychiatry, 29,* 11–20.

Rutter, M. (1988). Attention deficit disorder/hyperkinetic syndrome: Conceptual and research issues regarding diagnosis and classification. In T. Sagvolden & T. Archer (Eds.), *Attention deficit disorders and hyperkinetic syndrome.* Hillsdale, NJ: Erlbaum.

Satterfield, J., Hoppe, C.M., & Schell, A.M. (1982). A prospective study of delinquency in 110 adolescent boys with attention deficit disorder and 88 normal adolescent boys. *American Journal of Psychiatry, 139,* 795–798.

Scarr, S., & McCartney, K. (1985). How people make their own environments: A theory of genotype-environment effects. *Child Development, 54,* 424–435.

Schachar, R., Taylor, E., Wieselberg, M., Thorley, G., & Rutter, M. (1987). Changes in family function and relationships in children who respond to methylphenidate. *Journal of the American Academy of Child Psychiatry, 26,* 728–732.

Schmidt, M.H., Esser, G., Allehoff, W., Geisel, B., Laucht, M., & Woerner, W. (1987). Evaluating the significance of minimal brain dysfunction—Results of an epidemiological study. *Journal of Child Psychology and Psychiatry, 26,* 803–822.

Shen, Y.-C., Wong, Y.F., & Yang, X.L. (1985). An epidemiological investigation of minimal brain dysfunction in six elementary schools in Beijing. *Journal of Child Psychology and Psychiatry, 26,* 777–788.

Silva, P.A., Hughes, P., William, S., & Faed, V.M. (1988). Blood lead, intelligence, reading attainment, and behavior in 11-year-old children in Dunedin, New Zealand. *Journal of Child Psychology and Psychiatry, 29,* 43–52.

Taylor, E.A. (1986). Overactivity, hyperactivity and hyperkinesis: problems and prevalence. In E. A. Taylor (Ed.), *The overactive child. Clinics in developmental medicine,* No. 97. London: Mac Keith Press/Oxford: Blackwell.

Taylor, E.A. (1988 a). Attention deficit and conduct disorder syndromes. In M. Rutter, A. H. Tuma & I. S. Lann (Eds.), *Assessment and diagnosis in child psychopathology.* New York: Guilford Press.

Taylor, E.A. (1988 b). *An epidemiological study of childhood hyperactivity.* Research Report to the Medical Research Council.

Weiss, G., & Hechtman, L.T. (1986). *Hyperactive children grown up.* New York: Guilford.

Werry, J.S., Reeves, J.C., & Elkind, G.S. (1987). Attention deficit, conduct, oppositional and anxiety disorders in children: I. A review of research on differentiating characteristics; II. Clinical characteristics. *Journal of the American Academy of Child Psychiatry, 26,* 133–155.

Internalizing Disorders: Subtyping Based on Parental Questionnaires

Thomas M. Achenbach*

Because I was asked to focus on specific research results concerning internalizing disorders and because the time is so limited, I will report on the results of a body of research designed to test the replicability of a variety of empirically derived internalizing syndromes. I use the term "syndrome" here merely in its generic sense of a group of problems that tend to co-occur.

I would like to report findings in some detail, as we have just obtained them after several years of work and they are not available anywhere else. I will focus on the internalizing syndromes, but if time allows will also highlight some contrasts with externalizing syndromes derived in the same fashion. The findings are based on collaborative work with Professor Frank Verhulst, Director of Child Psychiatry at Sophia Children's Hospital, Rotterdam, Professor Keith Conners of Children's Hospital National Medical Center in Washington, D.C., and Professor Herbert Quay of the University of Miami, Florida.

Most diagnostic categories for adult psychiatric disorders had their origins in the 19th and early 20th centuries. Over several decades, efforts have been made to evolve more explicit and reliable research diagnostic criteria for the taxonomic constructs implied by the adult categories. Diagnostic categories for childhood disorders are much more recent, however, and they have not been refined through the development of research diagnostic criteria.

The lack of well-established diagnostic categories for childhood disorders has stimulated efforts to derive syndromes empirically through multivariate analyses of behavioral and emotional problems reported for children. Reviews of this research have revealed descriptive similarities among versions of syndromes obtained in multiple studies, despite differences in the subject samples, rating instruments, and methods of analysis (Achenbach, 1985; Achenbach & Edelbrock, 1978; Quay, 1986).

* This research was supported by the American Psychological Foundation and NIMH Grant MH40305. The author is grateful to Catherine T. Howell for her extensive analyses of the data.

The research that I will report was designed to provide more rigorous tests of the replicability of empirically derived syndromes and to yield firm operational definitions of the core syndromes. Such research is especially crucial for determining what so-called "internalizing" disorders actually exist, because "internalizing" problems are typically more subtle, variable, and less annoying to others than are the more easily identified "externalizing" behaviors. I will report findings for ages 6 to 16, although similar strategies are feasible for younger children and older adolescents, as well.

Methods

The data consisted of parents' ratings of three large multicenter samples of children referred to mental health services. As summarized in Table 1, the first sample consisted of 1,800 children referred to 42 different mental health services in the eastern United States during the 1970s (Achenbach & Edelbrock, 1981, 1983). Parents completed the *Child Behavior Checklist* (abbreviated CBCL), which consists of 20 social competence items and 118 items describing behavioral and emotional problems that are scored 0 if *not true* of the child, 1 if *somewhat or sometimes true,* and 2 if *very true or often true.*

The second sample consisted of 1,931 children referred to 17 mental health services in the Netherlands during the 1980s (Achenbach et al., 1987; Verhulst et al., 1988). Their parents completed a Dutch translation of the CBCL.

The third sample consisted of 4,481 children referred to 18 clinical services distributed throughout the United States in the

Table 1. Sources of data for testing the replicability of empirically derived syndromes.

---

1. *American Child Behavior Checklist (CBCL) Sample*
    1,800 6- to 16-year-olds seen in 42 mental health services in the eastern United States during the 1970s
2. *Dutch Child Behavior Checklist Sample*
    1,931 6- to 16-year-olds seen in 17 mental health services in the Netherlands during the 1980s
3. *American ACQ Behavior Checklist Sample*
    4,481 6- to 16-year-olds seen in 18 mental health services distributed across the United States during the 1980s

---

NOTE: Separate analyses were performed for all 215 ACQ problem items and for the ACQ counterparts of 115 CBCL items.

1980s. Their parents completed the *ACQ Behavior Checklist*, which was developed by Herbert Quay, Keith Conners, and myself to test the replicability of syndromes hypothesized on the basis of all the previous multivariate studies. The ACQ includes counterparts of 115 of the 118 CBCL problem items, plus an additional 100 problem items. The ACQ problem items are scored 0 for *never or not at all true*, 1 for *once in a while or just a little*, 2 for *quite often or quite a lot*, and 3 for *very often or very much*. Because 115 of the CBCL items have counterparts on the ACQ, we did separate analyses of this subset of 115 ACQ items as well as the entire set of 215 ACQ items.

For those of you who are interested in the statistical methodology, I will briefly summarize some technical details before presenting substantive findings and conclusions.

For each sample, principal components analyses were performed on item scores separately for children grouped by each sex within the age ranges 6 to 11 and 12 to 16 years. As summarized in Table 2, there were thus 16 separate principal components analyses. Varimax rotations were applied to each of the components analyses to identify the syndromes that were most robust in each source of data. Syndromes were operationally defined as the items loading highest in the varimax rotation that was retained for each group.

Table 2. Samples subjected to 16 principal components analyses with varimax rotations.

American CBCL
  1. Boys 6–11 (N = 450)   3. Boys 12–16 (N = 450)
  2. Girls 6–11 (N = 450)   4. Girls 12–16 (N = 450)
Dutch CBCL
  5. Boys 6–11 (N = 504)   7. Boys 12–16 (N = 461)
  6. Girls 6–11 (N = 530)   8. Girls 12–16 (N = 418)
American ACQ, all items
  9. Boys 6–11 (N = 1,750)   11. Boys 12–16 (N = 954)
 10. Girls 6–11 (N = 1,088)   12. Girls 12–16 (N = 689)
American ACQ, subset of CBCL items
 13. Boys 6–11 (N = 1,750)   15. Boys 12–16 (N = 954)
 14. Girls 6–11 (N = 1,088)   16. Girls 12–16 (N = 689)

For each sex within each age range, we thus obtained a score for each of four analyses a set of empirically derived syndromes. We then sought to answer the following question: How concordant are the different versions of a particular syndrome when applied to the same children (see Table 3)?

Table 3.

Question: How concordant are the different versions of a syndrome when
   applied to the same children?
Quantitative answer: Compute correlations between the four versions of
   each syndrome scored for the ACQ subjects.
   NOTE: Syndrome score = sum of the scores (0,1,2,3) for all items of a
   syndrome, as scored on the ACQ.
Core version of each syndrome: The items that were found in 3 or more
   components analyses for each sex/age group.
*Precaution to subtract general pathology from correlations between
   syndromes:* Partial out scores on nonsyndromal ACQ items from
   correlations between versions of a syndrome.

We obtained a quantitative index of the concordance between
syndromes in the following way: Because the *ACQ Behavior
Checklist* contained virtually all the items of the American and
Dutch versions of the CBCL as well as 100 additional items,
and because the samples were largest for the ACQ, we computed a score for each ACQ subject on the items comprising
each version of a syndrome for that subject's age and sex.

As an example, consider the 1,750 6- to 11-year-old boys
whose parents had completed ACQs in 18 different mental
health services. For each of these boys, we first added up their
scores of 0, 1, 2, and 3 on each item of each syndrome obtained
from the rotated principal components of the entire ACQ item
set. Each boy thus obtained for each syndrome derived from the
entire ACQ item set. Second, we computed each boy's score on
the syndrome derived from the principal components analysis
of the subset of 115 CBCL items that are on the ACQ. Third,
we computed each boy's score on the ACQ items corresponding
to those of the syndromes derived from the Dutch CBCL.
Fourth, we computed each boy's score on the ACQ items corresponding to those of the syndromes derived from the American
CBCL. And finally, we constructed a *core version* of each syndrome. This core version consisted of all items that were included in at least three of the other four versions of the syndrome. We also computed each boy's score on the ACQ items
corresponding to the core syndrome.

We thus obtained up to five versions of each syndrome. To
quantify the concordance between the different versions of each
syndrome, we then computed Pearson correlations between all
the boys' scores on all five versions of a syndrome. The correlations tell us how strongly the boys' standing on each version
of the syndrome is associated with their standing on each of the

other versions of the syndrome. If the various versions of a syndrome correlate highly with each other, this supports the replicability of the syndrome. If the empirically derived versions also correlate highly with the core syndrome, this means that the core syndrome can serve as a good operational definition of the taxonomic construct that each of the various versions approximates.

In computing the correlations between syndromes, we took the following precaution: Because most measures of child psychopathology correlate positively with each other—just as measures of intelligence also correlate positively with each other—we subtracted the effect of general psychopathology from the correlations between each syndrome. We did this by computing partial correlations between the versions of each syndrome, with the scores for all ACQ items not on those syndromes partialled out. In other words, we prevented the correlations between versions of a syndrome from being augmented by their mutual association with a general psychopathology factor.

Results

Internalizing Syndromes

Table 4 summarizes the mean correlations between versions of internalizing syndromes that replicated in at least three of four principal components analyses for at least two of the sex/age groups. Classification of syndromes as internalizing is based on previous second-order factor analyses which showed that these

Table 4. Partial correlations between versions of replicated internalizing syndromes.

| Syndromes | Mean partial r between versions | | | |
	Boys 6–11	Girls 6–11	Boys 12–16	Girls 12–16
Anxious/depressed	.94	.95	.87	.91
Schizoid	.62[a]	.60	.43	.61
Socially inept	.95	–	.77	–
Somatic	.95	.93	.91	.95
Withdrawn	.84	.90	.93[a]	.91

[a]Found in only 3/4 of the analyses for this sex/age group.

syndromes grouped together on a single second-order factor. The broad-band grouping formed by these syndromes contrasted with syndromes that loaded on another second-order factor to form a grouping designated as externalizing, because it encompassed aggressive, delinquent, and hyperactive behavior. The syndrome designated as *Socially Inept*, however, had a moderate correlation with the externalizing grouping as well as with the internalizing grouping in the second-order analyses. Because of its ambiguous status and because it replicated only for boys, I will not discuss it further here, nor will I discuss the *Schizoid* syndrome, which replicated rather poorly among the analyses within each sex/age group.

The three internalizing syndromes that replicated very strongly within all four of the sex/age groups are labeled in Table 4 as *Anxious/Depressed, Somatic,* and *Withdrawn.* As you can see, the mean correlations for versions of these syndromes ranged from .84 for the *Withdrawn* syndrome among 6- to 11-year-old boys, to .95 for the *Anxious/Depressed* syndrome among 6- to 11-year-old girls and the *Somatic* syndrome among 6- to 11-year-old boys and 11- to 16-year-old girls. Considering that all the correlations were reduced somewhat by partialling out scores on all items excluded from the syndrome being analyzed, these correlations show great similarity among the different versions of the syndromes.

The labels for the syndromes are merely intended to be descriptive summaries of the items that are common to the various versions of the syndromes. The labels are not intended to imply assumptions about the underlying causes of the different syndromes.

Table 5 lists abbreviated versions of the items found in the core internalizing syndromes for three or more of the four sex/age groups. Each core version of a syndrome included somewhat more items than are listed here as being common to the core versions for all sex/age groups. The differences between core syndromes from one group to another may represent true sex and age differences in the phenotypic syndromes, or may represent statistical fluctuations. However, considering the large and diverse samples, the differences in item pools, and the multiple gating criteria for retaining syndromes, the evidence for syndromes consisting of the problems listed in Table 5 is very strong. We are currently analyzing the distributions and discriminative power of syndrome scores to identify the most effective clinical cut-off points for each sex within each age range.

Table 5. Items found in core internalizing syndromes for 3 or more sex/age groups.

Anxious/depressed	Somatic	Withdrawn
Fearful, anxious	Aches, pains	Prefers to be alone
Fears school	Dizziness	Refuses to talk
Fears impulses	Headaches	Secretive
Feels unloved	Nausea	Self-conscious
Feels too guilty	Stomach aches	Shy, timid
Feels inferior/worthless	Vomiting	Stares into space
Feels persecuted		Underactive
Lonely		Unhappy, sad, depressed
Needs to be perfect		Withdrawn
Nervous, tense		
Self-conscious		
Unhappy, sad, depressed		
Worries		

Externalizing Syndromes

To provide a counterpoint to the internalizing syndromes, Table 6 summarizes the mean correlations between versions of externalizing syndromes that replicated in at least three of the four principal components analyses for at least one sex/age group. Two syndromes—designated as *Cruel* and *Sex Problems*—were found in three out of four components analyses only for girls. I will discuss only the three syndromes that were found quite consistently for both sexes in both age ranges. These were designated *Aggressive, Attention Deficit,* and *Delinquent.* Replication of the *Delinquent* syndrome was somewhat weak among

Table 6. Partial correlations between versions of replicated externalizing syndromes.

Syndromes	Mean partial r between versions			
	Boys 6–11	Girls 6–11	Boys 12–16	Girls 12–16
Aggressive	.97	.96	.96	.95
Attention deficit	.90	.95	.88	.89
Cruel	–	.84	–	.85
Delinquent	.91	.74[a]	.95	.93
Sex problems	–	.56[a]	–	–

[a]Found in only 3/4 of analyses for this sex/age group.

6- to 11-year-old girls, yielding a mean correlation of .74 among the three components analyses in which it was found. However, replication of all the other syndromes was very strong in all four components analyses for all groups. As you can see, the mean correlations ranged from .88 for the *Attention Deficit* syndrome among 12- to 16-year-old boys, to .97 for the *Aggressive* syndrome among 6- to 11-year-old boys.

Table 7. Items found in core externalizing syndromes for 3 or more sex/age groups.

Aggressive	Attention deficit	Delinquent
Argues	Acts too young	Alcohol, drugs[a]
Brags, boasts	Can't concentrate	Bad companions
Bullies	Can't sit still	Cheats, lies
Demands attention	Confused	Destroys others' things[a]
Disobedient at home	Daydreams	Destroys own things[a]
Doesn't feel guilty	Impulsive	Disobedient at school[a]
Easily jealous	Poor school work	Runs away from home[a]
Impulsive	Poor coordination,	Set fires[a]
Loud	clumsy	Steals at home
Screams	Stares into space	Steals outside home
Shows off		Truancy[a]
Starts fights		Vandalism[a]
Stubborn, irritable		
Sudden mood changes		
Sulks		
Swearing, obscenity		
Talks too much		
Teases		
Temper tantrums		

[a]Age- or sex-specific items found in core syndromes for only 1 age or sex.

Table 7 lists the items common to the core syndromes for the three externalizing syndromes that were found in all groups. As you can see, many items were common to the core *Aggressive* syndrome for the various groups. The *Delinquent* syndrome, on the other hand, contained several items that loaded on the syndrome for only one age group or one sex. As might be expected, use of alcohol and drugs, running away from home, and truancy were found in the core *Delinquent* syndrome for 12- to 16-year-olds of both sexes, but not for 6- to 11-year-olds of either sex. Destroying own things, destroying things belonging to others, firesetting, and vandalism, by contrast, were found in the core *Delinquent* syndrome for boys in both age ranges, but not for girls in either age group.

Conclusions

Our findings provide strong evidence for three internalizing syndromes and three externalizing syndromes in parents' reports on children of both sexes at ages 6 to 16, plus additional syndromes that are less general. Using large normative and clinical samples, we are now establishing cut-offs on the distributions of syndrome scores to provide operational definitions of clinical deviance for each syndrome. The limited time precludes extensive discussion of our findings. I would, however, like to list three important qualifications:

— *Qualification 1*. I realize that all the data I've presented originated with parents' ratings. This is not because we think that parents' ratings should be the sole source or even the decisive source of data in the assessment of children. We have done meta-analyses of correlations between many types of informants which show that the correlations between informants seeing children in different contexts average only about .28 (Achenbach et al., 1987). From this, we concluded that no single source of data—including parents, teachers, mental health workers, observers, or self-reports—is sufficient for the assessment of individual children. Data from multiple sources is always needed and will often reveal discrepancies that must be dealt with. Furthermore, our multivariate analyses of reports by other informants do not yield exactly the same syndromes as reports by parents, although there are many important similarities. Nevertheless, parents are typically the main source of data about their children. Parents also know their children across longer time periods and more situations than others do. And parents' views are crucial in determining what will be done about a child. Data obtained from parents must therefore provide one cornerstone for the assessment of child psychopathology and the taxonomy of childhood disorders. We plan to present findings on relations between syndromes obtained from parents and from other sources, including teachers, observers, interviewers, and self-reports.

— *Qualification 2*. The syndromes we obtained reflect statistical associations between phenotypic characteristics, as reported by parents of large samples of clinically referred children. These syndromes enable us to group children for research on differential etiology, course, responsiveness to treatment, prognosis, and epidemiology. The syndromes themselves do not imply a commitment to particular theories of the disorders such as environmental versus genetic.

— *Qualification 3.* We do not claim that the syndromes we found are the only ones possible for ages 6 to 16. The use of different items, different informants, different subjects, and different methods of analysis might reveal additional syndromes. However, we do have considerable confidence in the syndromes that have replicated well. We feel that our multi-center research can contribute significantly to efforts to advance our knowledge of child psychopathology on many fronts and in many locations.

References

Achenbach, T. M. (1985). *Assessment and taxonomy of child and adolescent psychopathology.* Newbury Park, CA: Sage.

Achenbach, T. M., & Edelbrock, C. (1978). The classification of child psychopathology: A review and analysis of empirical efforts. *Psychological Bulletin, 85,* 1275–1301.

Achenbach, T. M., & Edelbrock, C. (1981). Behavioral problems and competencies reported by parents of normal and disturbed children aged four to sixteen. *Monographs of the Society for Research in Child Development, 46,* Serial No. 188.

Achenbach, T. M., & Edelbrock, C. (1983). *Manual for the Child Behavior Checklist and Revised Child Behavior Profile.* Burlington, VT: University of Vermont Department of Psychiatry.

Achenbach, T. M., McConaughy, S. H., & Howell, C. T. (1987). Child/adolescent behavioral and emotional problems: Implications of cross-informant correlations for situation specificity. *Psychological Bulletin, 101,* 213–232.

Achenbach, T. M., Verhulst, F. C., Baron, G. D., & Althaus, M. (1987). A comparison of syndromes derived from the Child Behavior Checklist for American and Dutch boys aged 6–11 and 12–16. *Journal of Child Psychology and Psychiatry, 28,* 437–453.

Quay, H. C. (1986). Classification. In H. C. Quay & J. S. Werry (Eds.), *Psychopathological disorders of childhood* (3rd ed.) (pp. 1–42). New York: Wiley.

Verhulst, F. C., Achenbach, T. M., Althaus, M., & Akkerhuis, G. W. (1988). A comparison of syndromes derived from the Child Behavior Checklist for American and Dutch girls aged 6–11 and 12–16. *Journal of Child Psychology and Psychiatry, 29,* 879–895.

Classification in Child Psychiatry: A Critique of Approaches Based on Parental Questionnaires

Antony D. Cox

Professor Achenbach's paper arises from a very extensive research program. An important focus has been the development of a rational system of diagnostic classification based on empirical findings rather than armchair theorizing. The populations studied have been predominantly, but not exclusively, clinical, it being argued that non-referred children would not reveal syndromes of clinical seriousness. A variety of instruments and informants have been used, but the *Parent-Child Behavior Checklist* (CBCL) and its successor, the *ACQ Behavior Checklist* have been most frequently employed because parents are seen as the most crucial and reliable source of data. The questionnaires are usually, but not always, self-administered and require parents to report on their child, indicating in the CBCL whether—considering the past 6 months—statements about behavior are "not true," "somewhat or sometimes true," or "very true or often true." The ACQ applies to 2 months and uses a 4-point scale as opposed to a 3-point scale: parents choose between "never or not at all," "once in a while or just a little," "quite often or quite a lot," "very often or very much."

Using large clinical populations in Holland and the United States, Professor Achenbach has demonstrated that certain behaviors reported by parents on the questionnaire showed consistency in the manner in which they are associated statistically. The consistency has been shown by scoring children from one population on syndromes derived from other populations employing questionnaires with common or overlapping items. Professor Achenbach indicates the need to determine cut-offs in order to provide operational definitions of clinical deviance. He makes important qualifications: Only one source of data on each child has been employed, the syndromes are descriptive with no specific implications for etiology, and the syndromes obtained do not comprehend all possible syndromes.

It has been suggested that classification is vital to provide an agreed-upon, that is, *reliable* set of terms for accurate communication with respect to clinical assessments, research, and the monitoring and planning of services (Rutter & Gould, 1985). Therefore, classification based on idiosyncratic theory may have a function in research, but will not be useful in general clinical practice.

If a system of classification is to be useful, it must validly reflect current empirically derived knowledge. As such, it constitutes a series of hypotheses about distinctions between patterns of behavior which need to be tested for their capacity to discriminate relevantly with respect to the understanding of etiology, indications about intervention, and prognosis. Since reliability/agreement between clinicians is crucial, diagnostic terms require operational definitions. However, there must also be agreement on the quality and appropriateness of sources of data on which the diagnostic decisions are made.

Individual children may exhibit more than one pattern of behavior at any one time or at different times, so that classifications are of *disorders* not children. In childhood, account must be taken of development, including the possibility that onset of particular disorders may be peculiar to particular stages of development.

A classification should attempt to cover all patterns of disorder, be logically consistent, and practicable in clinical practice.

Professor Achenbach's paper is clearly and carefully constructed. I would like to ask questions about a number of minor matters and then address three more major issues.

Firstly: What difference does it make that some factor structures were derived from 3-point items and some from 4-point items? *Secondly*: What was the criterion for "loading highest"? Was this determined by the extent of loading, or rank order of loading? *Thirdly*: What would have happened if children's syndrome scores were obtained by adding items weighted according to the loading of the item for the syndrome in question? *Fourthly*: What difference does it make that the CBCL is scored for a 6-month period and the ACQ for 2 months? *Fifthly*: Could it be that analyses extract traits rather than states?

Now more major issues:

1. The approach to classification described by Professor Achenbach is reliable, is capable of operational definition, testable as regards validity, logically consistent, and practicable. Furthermore, it classifies disorders and not children, and aims to be responsive to developmental changes.

However, there are issues about the source of data used to derive the classification, the relevance of the discriminations to clinical practice, and comprehensiveness.

Consider the questionnaire instrument as a source of data for classification. Firstly, data is derived from only one source. Professor Achenbach has himself addressed this issue not only in his qualifications to the paper, but in proposing elsewhere the use of a multiaxial classification system in clinical practice, such that different axes reflect syndromes derived from data from different sources (Achenbach et al., 1987). Secondly, the questionnaire method does not allow informants interpretation or understanding of items to be tested. Thirdly, although the social competence items of the questionnaire could in some measure be used to assess severity or impact of the disorder, they do not appear to be used in this way in deciding what items enter the analyses. Fourthly, scales for individual items give points equal weight yet items differ in psychopathological significance and in their scaling. For example, the point "once in a while or just a little" may be important clinically for some items and not for others. Items certainly differ markedly in the extent to which they discriminate between clinical and non-clinical populations (Achenbach & Edelbrock, 1981). Some items refer to behavioral events, some to pervasive aspects of behavior, some to experiences that may vary in intensity, some that may vary in persistence, and some that may vary in frequency—in some cases high pathology might be indicated by low frequency and in others by high frequency.

Although the social competence items ask parents to calibrate according to age, it is not known how much parents adjust their own scaling according to the child's stage of development when scoring behavioral items. Are they scoring against absolute or normative criteria, taking into account the child's age and social circumstances? Fifthly, with regard to duration, the longer period over which parents rate with the CBCL may pick up chronic disorders or personality traits and underrepresent acute disorders, while the shorter duration ACQ may underrepresent recurrent disorders.

Use of a parental questionnaire as a data source is not a problem when it is needed as a screening instrument, as a method to explore broad patterning of behavior, or to raise hypotheses; but it is more questionable as a basis for diagnostic classification in clinical practice. In clinical practice, data from a wide range of sources are collated, checked, and weighed before a diagnosis is reached. In his proposal for a 5-axis diagnostic system, Professor Achenbach suggests one axis should encompass data from parents, one from teachers, and a third data from direct assessment using clinical interview, self-ratings, and observations. If data from all these sources are necessary for a good clinical assessment, shouldn't such data be the basis for empirically derived classification? Recent reports suggest that better discrimination between syndromes can be obtained when parent and teacher ratings on the Revised CBCL are combined (Mattison et al., 1987). Other reports indicate that semi-structured interviews with parent and child generate better agreement between informants than do questionnaires (Verhulst et al., 1987).

2. Turning to the mode of analysis, it has been suggested this places more emphasis on what characteristics children have in common and therefore does not pick out rare syndromes (Rutter & Gould, 1985) or those where there is only one symptom of very high or incapacitating severity. In other words, the approach does not lead to a comprehensive classification.

3. Finally I wish to refer to the need for classifications to adapt in the light of advancing knowledge. Disorders found in DSM-III-R and draft ICD 10 (Rutter, 1988) in comparison with DSM-III and ICD 9 include more whose defining criteria relate to development, relationships, and circumstances. These changes reflect research findings. Could questionnaire assessments be adapted to reflect research findings in a similar way? I understand the ACQ intended to do so in comparison with the CBCL, but that this then discriminated less well between clinical and non-clinical populations (Achenbach, 1988).

I suggest that the way forward in developing classification lies in using a combination of standardized instruments, whose measurements incorporate developmental and disability criteria, and which relate behavior to circumstances and relationships in ways that research suggests may discriminate usefully in regard to etiology, treatment, and prognosis. Examples of behavioral symptoms that are related to development, relationships, and circumstances are pervasive attentional difficulty, stealing from caretakers, destructiveness to objects as opposed to persons, separation anxiety, and post-traumatic flashbacks.

References

Achenbach, T. M., & Edelbrock, C. S. (1981). *Behavioral problems and competences reported by parents of normal and disturbed children aged four through sixteen.* Monographs of the Society of Research in Child Development, Vol. 46. No. 1.

Achenbach, T. M., McConaughy, S. H, & Howell, C. T. (1987). Child-adolescent behavioral and emotional problems: Implications of cross informant correlations for situation specificity. *Psychological Bulletin, 101,* 213–232.

Achenbach, T. M. (1988). Personal communication.

American Psychiatric Association (1987). *Diagnostic and statistical manual of mental disorders* (3rd ed., rev.). Washington: Author.

Mattison, R. E., Bagnato, S. J., & Strickler, E. (1987). Diagnostic importance of combined parent and teacher ratings on the *Revised Behavior Problem Check-List. Journal of Abnormal Child Psychology, 15,* 617–628.

Rutter, M., & Gould, M. (1985). Classification (Chapter 18). In M. Rutter & L. Hersov (Eds.), *Child and adolescent psychiatry: Modern approaches* (pp. 305–321). Oxford: Blackwell.

Rutter, M. (1988). ICD 10. Personal Communication.

Verhulst, F. C., Althaus, M., & Burden, G. F. M. G. (1987). The *Child Assessment Schedule*: Parent-child-agreement and validity measures. *Journal of Child Psychology and Psychiatry, 28,* 455–466.

Disorders Related to Maturational Problems

Joest Martinius

The three groups of disorders to be dealt with in this paper are very different from each other, each of them related to maturation but each in different ways. To group them together is therefore somewhat arbitrary. Enuresis and encopresis have in common that they are the expression of disordered processes of retention and elimination, and that their presence may—and in the case of encopresis always does—cause serious detriments to social and psychic well-being, whereas speech disorders primarily interfere with communication and are not necessarily detrimental to well-being. Disordered processes of elimination and speech disorders have strong links to maturation. Sleep disorders in children are somewhat less obvious. They usually are very disturbing to the family but not so much to the child or to the social environment other than the family, and in their majority are not directly related to maturation. Only distinct entities such as night terrors and sleep-walking are clearly problems of maturation.

Research on these problems in Germany has been and is, with the exception perhaps of speech problems, not very active. This statement pertains to child psychiatry as well as to pediatrics. This fact is the more surprising since all these problems occur frequently at given ages, letting many children suffer considerably. The limited interest in doing research may have several reasons, about which one can only speculate. Most certainly one reason is the fact that disorders related to maturation have a tendency to improve spontaneously with ongoing maturation and eventually to disappear. Second, maturation is a physical process linked to neural substrates, central and peripheral, that are difficult to study on a neuronal level, particularly in children. And third, fashionable beliefs exist that are misleading or even obviously wrong though nevertheless passed on and perpetuated with great conviction. It is still widely held, for instance, that disorders of elimination are purely psychogenic in origin, and that the only successful method of dealing with them is the corresponding model of psychotherapy. The unfortunate consequence of such an undifferentiated standpoint is the assumption that all answers have already been given and that no further research is needed.

Disorders of the Processes of Retention and Elimination

Enuresis

Enuresis is a symptom. Its causation is rarely unidirectional, as is the case with urinary tract anomalies and infections. The distinction between primary and secondary forms on the basis of an interval of complete control for six months is useful though not sufficient for research purposes. Yet, there still are studies undertaken that define enuretic children only by the presence of the symptom. Such studies are at best replicating known facts and are thus scientifically useless. Since much is known about factors contributing to etiology, research will have to concentrate upon these factors in order to study subgroups of better defined enuretic children and to compare these groups (Table 1). Thereby we should come to the position of clearly

Table 1. Pathogenetic factors associated with enuresis (Gross & Dornbusch, 1983).

Genetic
Demographic
    Socioeconomic status
    Family size
    Birth order
Maturational delay
    Birth weight
    Bone age
    Motor delay
    Sexual
Psychosocial
    Stress, emotional disturbance
    Behavioral deviance
    Toilet training
Sleep disturbance
Psychiatric disorders
Organic
    Urinary tract infection
    Lumbosacral anomalies
    Diabetes mellitus
    Insipidus

identifying children with maturational delay, those with adverse psychosocial circumstances, and those with other major contributing influences. Subgroups of enuretic children should be studied longitudinally, carefully specifying the frequency and nature of wetting and of maturational parameters at each age in the developing child so that the dependent variable can be recognized reliably, i.e., secondary or primary. Maturational parameters would have to include neurophysiological measures. Along with these, stressful social conditions, family structure, and patterns of family interaction have to be recorded carefully, a task child psychiatrists are well trained to accomplish. A longitudinal study with an early beginning would also be the proper approach for answering the most interesting question of whether there is a sensitive period for toilet training. The results of the kibbutz study by Kaffman and Elizur (1977) are very suggestive in this direction: Toilet training was facilitated when begun between 12 and 15 months and retarded when begun after 20 months of age.

The factorial model calls for an individualized combination of elective treatments. Properly evaluated methods are available. What happens in practice, however, presents a different picture. Diverse opinions reflected in the literature and actual professional behavior give evidence of a general confusion, composed of ideologies and ignorance. Research could be very useful in the form of surveys, evaluating the present situation of enuretic children as well as professional and nonprofessional methods of intervention and support. The aim of such studies would be the establishment of educational programs for people working in the health field.

Encopresis

The situation with encopresis is different in some aspects. Encopresis occurs less frequently (1.5% of the 8-year-olds), shows an even greater preponderance in boys, shows no social class preference and no indication that prevalence relates to family size, ordinal position, or age of parents (Levine, 1975). The symptom constitutes a functional disturbance of bowel motility. The pathophysiologic processes initiating the symptom are not thoroughly understood. The view is maintained that constitutional and/or acquired derangements of bowel motility induce vulnerability to encopresis and that psychogenic and sociogenic traumata lead to manifestation of the disease. A maturational background is to be postulated since bowel control is normally acquired by maturation and training, and since cases of primary encopresis can be seen (Olatawura, 1973). The distinction between primary and secondary encopresis is, however, even less clear than in enuresis. Basic research is needed to learn more about maturation of bowel motility and about pathophysiological mechanisms altering it, setting the ground for retention and accumulation of fecal material. This type of study has technical and psychological implications and requires the cooperation of pediatric surgeons, pediatricians, and psychiatrists.

Even more than in enuresis the notion is still held that a distinct parental (maternal) personality and abnormal processes of family interaction are primary if not exclusive causes for the development of encopresis in the child. One more recent German study failed to confirm the traditional position (mainly held by psychoanalysts) (Artner & Castell, 1981). Nevertheless, with an encopretic child, family interaction is soon disturbed, the child becoming emotionally disturbed. These interactional processes need further clarification, at best in a multicenter study in order to collect a representative number of families and to follow them at least over a decade. Intervention can be reevaluated and long-term prognosis described.

According to Levine and Bakow (1976), about 20% of encopretic children show resistance to the established multimodal treatment, i.e., bowel training, family counseling, and individual psychotherapy. This particular group of children needs further study.

Encopresis is odorous, and perhaps there is a psychological barrier, impeding research in this area. Most important are basic studies on pathophysiology and evaluation studies.

Speech Disorders

Speech development is tied closely to the maturation of the central nervous system. There is an anatomical functional basis for speech in the form of hemisphere specialization, which appears to be inborn. Consequently, if brain maturation is altered in one or another way, there is a great likelihood for the development of speech to be disturbed as well. Along with the discovery of techniques for the study of neural structure and function, strong impulses have been given to correlative studies of brain dysfunction and developmental language disorders. Child psychiatry has traditionally and actively performed research in this area, particularly with regard to the developmental aphasias or specific language disabilities, respectively, the clinical problems ranging anywhere between early infantile autism on the one and dyslexia on the other end of the list.

But there is the danger now that child psychiatry in this country is not keeping step with the research standards met elsewhere. Because so many clinical departments have totally subscribed to psychotherapeutic work, and even some university departments have never paid much attention to neurophysiological techniques such as the recording of evoked potentials or brain mapping, only few laboratories exist in child psychiatric clinics in which correlative neurophysiological and neuropsychological research can be done.

The first research requirement in the area of speech disorders is the study of the *normal* development of speech. The prespeech period is of prime interest. Very active research has been made and is going on at the Max Planck Institute for Psychiatry in Munich (Papousek & Papousek, 1986), now threatened by loss of funding. Another active research group at the same institute is investigating motor aspects of speech production in children with developmental language problems, using phonological techniques (Amorosa et al., 1988). The latter group has produced clear evidence that phonation sonograms are excellent measures for speech–motor coordination and its disturbances. The future of this group is uncertain as well.

Research of this type is basic, though the results have immediate practical implications, since an improved knowledge about motor aspects of speech production can be translated into new therapeutic approaches. The importance of studying early communicative processes, including preverbal vocal interaction is obvious.

Within the entire field of speech disorders, several of the areas in which research needs to be done or needs to be intensified are of prime importance. These are speech perception and comprehension, articulation, syntax, and, finally, the social communicative aspects of language in their normal and disturbed appearances. We should, for instance, come into the position to predict reliably and quantitatively at the end of the second year of life in a given child the risk for a speech disorder. Again, longitudinal investigations are necessary, incorporating audiologic, neuromotor, linguistic, and neuropsychological research potentials. This would be a major project that would have to be initiated regionally where the specific faculties mentioned are in close contact to each other. One of the various questions such a study could deal with is that of the relationship between language development and cognitive development. Another question is whether compensatory nonverbal communicative skills in children with speech disorders may or may not develop and in which way psychic development is affected. Speech disorders in children are an important field for research carrying a large potential for future expansion. Child psychiatry is well advised to engage actively in this field.

Sleep Disorders

Many children have sleep problems, the majority of which is reactive in nature and relatively easy to remedy by changing parent–child interaction. But a significant number of children suffer in a stricter sense from sleep disturbances originating from deviant maturational processes in the brain. These are:

— disorders of excessive somnolence (*hypersomnias*);

— disorders of initiating and maintaining sleep (*insomnias*);

— dysfunctions associated with sleep, sleep stages, or partial arousal (*parasomnias*);

— disorders of sleep–wake schedule (*phase lag syndromes*).

The regulation of sleep is profoundly correlated with maturation of the central nervous system. Sleep disorder evaluations require the study of 24-hour diurnal organization of waking and sleep behavior and of biorhythmic functions of body systems (autonomic, sensorimotor, neuroendocrine). In the past three decades sleep disorder medicine has emerged as a new field. Again, in Germany, research in this field has been largely neglected in children, with the exception of studies in newborns and young infants. Consequently, knowledge is restricted, respective chapters in textbooks are missing or antiquated, and the care of children and adolescents with sleep disturbances is rather incidental. The reason for this deplorable situation may be the high technical, temporal, and personal expenditures that are required. On the other hand, there is definitely the need for doing research on sleep disorders, relating maturation, measured by neurophysiological parameters, to the functional disturbance—for instance, night terrors and sleep-walking—and learning more about emotional influences upon the occurrence of these disturbances. There are questions common to child psychiatry and child neurology concerning the organization of sleep in disease processes affecting the central nervous system, traumatic and progressive. And finally, sleep research similar to that performed in psychiatry on adult psychotic patients is overdue in child and adolescent psychiatry.

The younger a child is, the closer behavioral and emotional disturbances are entangled with maturation. The few entities dealt with in this presentation are only examples out of a larger collection. Child and adolescent psychiatry is subjected to episodic changes of preferred areas of interest. Maturation has, in recent years, occupied a subordinate position in relation to psychosocial influences upon development and developmental problems.

I hope to have stimulated the will to rearrange research activities into proper proportions.

References

Amorosa, H., von Benda, U., & Wagner, E. (1988). Voice problems in children with unintelligible speech as indicators of deficits in fine motor coordination. *Folia phoniatrica*, in press.

Artner, K., & Castell, R. (1981). Enkopresis-Diagnostik und stationäre Therapie. In Ch. Steinhausen (Ed.), *Psychosomatische Störungen und Krankheiten bei Kindern und Jugendlichen*. Stuttgart: Kohlhammer.

Gross, R. T., & Dornbusch, S. M. (1983). Disordered processes of elimination: enuresis. In R. T. Gross (Ed.), *Developmental behavioral pediatrics*. Philadelphia: Saunders Co.

Kaffman, M., & Elizur, E. (1977). Infants who become enuretics: A longitudinal study of 161 kibbutz-children. *Monographs of the Society of Research in Child Development, 42*, 2–23.

Levine, M. D. (1975). Children with encopresis: A descriptive analysis. *Paediatrics, 56*, 412–416.

Levine, M. D., & Bakow, H. (1976). Children with encopresis: A study of treatment outcome. *Pediatrics, 58*, 845–852.

Olatawura, M. O. (1973). Encopresis, a review of 32 cases. *Acta Paediatrica Scandinavica, 62*, 358–364.

Papousek, H., & Papousek, M. (1986). Structure and dynamics of human communication at the beginning of life. *European Archive of Psychiatry and Neurological Sciences, 236*, 21–25.

A Closer Look at Maturational Factors

Aribert Rothenberger

Maturational Delay vs Maturational Deviation

Professor Martinius gave us a well-guided survey of the topic. Allow me to present here a closer look at neuronal maturational factors, which seem to be a central point for this issue.

In principle, we agree with Professor Martinius that each of the disorders mentioned seems to have a neuronal maturational problem (or more generally: developmental problem), and that we should try to find out in more detail the pathophysiological basis of these maturational problems. If we do so, we should be aware of two aspects of maturational problems: the distinction between maturational delay and maturational deviation.

A true maturational delay detected in a child at a certain age means that the registered value of that parameter can be defined as normal in a significantly younger child. In contrast, a maturational deviation means that the data of a certain child deviate from the characteristics of all the normal values along the developmental axis.

For example, an occipital alpha-theta ratio (ATR, a matter of change, but with high reliability over time) of two in the EEG of a 13-year-old is not adequate for that age—it should be around four (8-year-olds normally have an ATR of two). Thus, the finding in this child reflects a *maturational delay.* But if we find graphoelements like vertex transients or occipital transients and a fair amount of non-drug-induced beta-spindles in a child's waking EEG record (matters with high stability over time), then we can assume a *maturational deviation,* since these EEG signs usually do not occur during normal development of electrical brain activity.

It is not uncommon to detect both maturational delay and maturational deviation within the same EEG record of a child, and it is certainly not rare that a maturational delay recovers completely over time. The so-called persisting maturational delay has to be kept in mind, too.

Another example can be given with respect to the behaviorally defined soft neurological signs. Involuntary mirror movements can be seen very often in younger children, but they decrease in frequency as the children get older. When this behavior is detected as a motor abnormality in older children, it reflects a maturational delay either persisting in the future or decreasing to adequate age-related behavior in due time. On the other hand, nonphysiologic nystagmus (e.g., fixation nystagmus) clearly reflects a maturational deviation and has little chance to disappear later on.

Call for Longitudinal Studies

Most of our knowledge about maturational problems in child psychiatry comes from cross-sectional studies. Yet they give no valid information about the true maturation of individuals or child psychiatric groups over time—and just that is what is needed at different investigational levels to detect and evaluate maturational factors of prognostic value for daily clinical practice. Thus, in the research field of dyslexia, dysphasia, sleeping disorders, enuresis, and others, longitudinal studies of well-defined groups (and not necessarily only subgroups) have to be conducted for a successful approach to the specific maturational problems involved in these disorders.

Appropriate methods for such longitudinal studies are available. As we could show at the neurophysiological level, EEG power spectra and evoked potentials have a good test-retest reliability over long time spans (Rothenberger et al., 1987; Woerner et al., 1987). At the neuropsychological level, test performance was also quite stable over time (Woerner & Rothenberger, 1985). Most of the children entered a certain maturational level within their age group and developed along this level (percentile). Only a few children changed this level over time to become better or worse.

Brain Maturation and Behavior

In the research on maturational problems the question of whether or not there is a causal relationship between the central nervous maturational status and observed behavior plays an important role. The long debate focusing on minimal cerebral damage (Schmidt et al., 1987) can easily be transferred to the disorders we are talking about here. Certainly, no one would contradict the statement that all human behavior is regulated by the central nervous system (CNS). Nevertheless, modern methods, including the brand-new imaging techniques such as PET and MRI, do not give full insight into brain functioning. Therefore, it is not surprising that there is no 100% correlation between available basic CNS data at the neuro-chemical, neurophysiological, and neuropsychological level on the one hand, and psychopathological behavior on the other. In addition, we have to take into consideration that a certain deficit of the central nervous maturational status which would usually lead to behavioral disturbance may be compensated at the behavioral level by other functional neuronal networks of the brain. We know this from work with aphasic children (Rothenberger, 1986).

Maturational Aspects of Some Child Psychiatric Disorders

In *externalizing disorders* the very low alpha-theta ratio of the EEG at age 8 can mature rapidly until age 13 and reach almost normal values, although other EEG signs like deviant gra-phoelements may remain stable over time; additionally, exter-nalizers may approach normal amplitude values of evoked po-tentials from age 8 to 13. Those who fail to show this electrophysiological after-maturation may have a somewhat higher risk for behavioral disturbances (Rothenberger & Woerner, 1986).

For normal and pathological development of *speech and lan-guage*, the old hypothesis of a different maturation of both hemispheres should be reevaluated, since new techniques of topographical EEG analysis allow a better regional resolution of left/right and anterior/posterior direction. In addition, recent large-scale studies of EEG power spectra, phase, and coherence across the developmental span show distinct patterns of age-related development for left and right cerebral hemispheres. The growth spurt of the left hemisphere at age 4–6 appears to coincide with milestones of cognitive and linguistic development (Thatcher et al., 1987; Rothenberger et al., 1984). Furthermore,

Jernigan et al. (1987) have reported preliminary results from MRI studies of language-impaired and control children: Whereas all five of the control children scanned had a larger left than right posterior region of the brain, six of the ten language-impaired children had a larger right than left posterior region. These six children also had a decrease in gray matter and an increase in fluid in these brain regions.

The step to define the basic maturational deficits in language-impaired children should be followed by a closely related topic: the question of how a well-known brain status can be functionally optimized by environmental stimulation. That a nonoptimal timing between brain and environment leads to low behavioral performance of the child can be seen in deprived children like Kaspar Hauser or Geenie (Rothenberger, 1986). For a child with a maturational deficit, a mismatch—too high or too low in quantity, wrong in quality—between inner and outer world can be unfavorable. Thus, the efficiency of our treatments depends, among other things, on our knowledge of the child's brain status.

For *sleeping disorders*, we have a good chance to obtain more insight into, and an understanding of, the basic maturational brain mechanisms. Polygraphic recordings in a longitudinal setting from age 3 to 10 could give us more detailed information on normal and abnormal development of sleep organization in children. Especially the crucial role of the arousal reaction from slow-wave sleep to REM sleep has to be investigated in more depth. We know very little about the influences of the many hours of brain activity during children's sleep in relation to child psychiatric disorders. For children with parasomnias, the REM-arousal mechanism as well as the neuronal discoupling between peripheral and central motor systems during REM phases seem to be immature (Rothenberger, 1988).

Finally, neuronal maturational deficits seem to play an important role in *enuretic children* who may have a high CNS detection level for autonomic signals of their body, probably in the sense of an autonomic neuropathy known from diabetics. One could also follow up on the question of whether there is a mismatch between the peripheral urodynamic bladder function and the central nervous coordination of the whole evacuation process. There is a great interest among pediatric urologists and sleep researchers to cooperate with child psychiatrists on studies like this.

Conclusion

There are many more interesting—and not only neuronal—maturational problems in child psychiatric disorders to solve than I could present. If we were to initiate further research in this area, we could, with some effort, develop a better basis for the understanding of the disorder-specific neuronal weakness (locus minoris resistentiae, specific vulnerability), its interaction with the unspecific environmental stress factors, and the compensatory factors within and without a child's brain. In this manner we may be able to work out more efficient treatments for child psychiatric patients.

References

Jernigan, T. L., Hesselink, J., & Tallal, P. (1987). Cerebral morphology on magnetic resonance imaging in developmental dysphasia. *Soc. Neurosci. Abstr., 13*(1), 651.

Rothenberger, A. (1986). Aphasie bei Kindern. *Fortschritte der Neurologie und Psychiatrie, 54*, 92–98.

Rothenberger, A. (1988). Somnambulismus and Pavor nocturnus—Knotenpunkte in einem Verhaltensspektrum. *Pädiatrische Praxis* (in press).

Rothenberger, A., & Woerner, W. (1986). Elektrische Hirnaktivität bei kinderpsychiatrischen Störungen im Längsschnitt von 8 bis 13 Jahren—Eine epidemiologische Studie. In M. H. Schmidt & S. Drömann (Eds.), *Langzeitverlauf kinder- und jugendpsychiatrischer Erkrankungen* (pp. 91–98). Stuttgart: Enke.

Rothenberger, A., Woerner, W., & Blanz, B. (1987). Test-retest reliability of flash-evoked potentials in a field sample: A 5 year follow-up in school children with and without psychiatric disturbances. In R. Johnson, Jr., J. W. Rohrbough, & R. Parasuraman (Eds.), *Current trends in event-related potential research* (pp. 624–628) (Electroencephalography and clinical neurophysiology, Suppl. 40).

Schmidt, M. H., Esser, G., Allehoff, W., Geisel, B., Laucht, M., & Woerner, W. (1987). Evaluating the significance of minimal brain dysfunction—Results of an epidemiological study. *Journal of Child Psychology and Psychiatry, 6*, 803–821.

Thatcher, R. W., Walker, R. A., & Giudice, S. (1987). Human cerebral hemispheres develop at different rates and ages. *Science, 236*, 1110–1113.

Woerner, W., & Rothenberger, A. (1985). EEG power spectra and psychometric test performance at ages 8 and 13. A longitudinal study. *International Journal of Psychophysiology, 2*, 217.

Woerner, W., Rothenberger, A., & Lahnert, B. (1987). Test-retest reliability of spectral parameters of the resting EEG in a field sample: A 5 year follow-up in school children with and without psychiatric disturbances. In R. Johnson, Jr., J. W. Rohrbough, & R. Parasuraman (Eds.), *Current trends in event-related potential research* (pp. 629–632) (Electroencephalography and clinical neurophysiology, Suppl. 40).

SECTION III:

PERSPECTIVES OF INTERVENTION RESEARCH

Epidemiology: Perspectives of Future Research

Martin H. Schmidt

Epidemiology is one of those subfields of child and adolescent psychiatry that has experienced an intensive development during the last 20 years, and at the same time it is one of those fields in which a couple of questions concerning both substance and methodology seem to be, at least for the time being, satisfactorily solved. Nevertheless, there still are a number of problems left open. I will refer mainly to these "gaps of knowledge" and by doing so I do not mean to play down the progress achieved and the scientists involved therein.

Problems of Case Definition and Identification

Let me start with methodological questions, to be more exact: problems of case definition. It is generally agreed today that case definition should not—as far as possible—be grounded neither upon single symptoms nor on a sum of symptoms, ideally not even solely on statistically derived dimensions of deviant behavior (as systematically developed by Achenbach, 1985), but rather on diagnoses concerning aberrant behavior that demands intervention. Such diagnoses have to be assignable to rough categories of disease.

Ideally these diagnoses should be completed by the given grade of severity that informs about the need of treatment and the necessary therapeutic efforts. Given this information, it would be possible to compare patient samples differing with respect to the efforts they demand. Even now it is rather impossible to compare grades of severity; there are scarcely any methods for comparisons within one diagnostic category, let alone any at all for a comparison between diagnostic categories.

Where an estimation is desired of how much a disorder does damage to the development potential of a child, that is to say, where both a prognosis of the course of disease and of the normal pace of development is wanted, an even broader case definition is required. We know forms of disorder, for example, schizophrenia of disintegrative or hebephrenic type, that finally call for pedagogical rather than intensive psychotherapeutic effort, but have a drastic effect on the patient's life quality, and vice versa. What we therefore need are additional indicators of the adaptive potential of patients or their ability to manage developmental tasks. Full adaptation can be attained after recovery or only partial recovery, as is the case in impairments. Such information is in particular necessary in all designs in which cohorts of both disturbed and undisturbed children/adolescents are examined. All propositions in existence for measuring the adaptive level (e.g., Shaffer et al., 1983) are unsatisfactory, as they are not really one-dimensional; they combine residual or non-affected abilities of the patient with symptoms on a one-dimensional continuum.

Epidemiological research is concentrated on identifying protective or pathogenic factors rather than mechanisms or processes. These, however, are crucial for a deeper understanding of how adaptation/maladaptation develops. The absence of negative influences cannot per se be seen as having a protective effect, and the mere presence of "protective" influences does not necessarily have a buffering effect leading to adaptation. Protection and vulnerability are not just two sides of one coin; reversibility is not automatically given. We need to think of so-called "catalytic factors" (Rutter, 1985), that is, factors "that are largely inert on their own but, when combined with environmental stresses or hazards, either increase their effect (so-called 'vulnerability' factors), or decrease their impact (so-called 'protective' factors)" (Rutter, 1985, p. 390). The presence of a supportive social network, for example, is thought to operate in that way. Allowing for such catalytic effects leads to very complex models.

Case definition of psychiatric syndromes in the narrow sense does not face the same difficulties. Because of the necessity of epidemiological studies to differentiate not only between "healthy" and "deviant," but even within the range of normality, and because of the rarity of extremely pathological findings, it is not appropriate to use the same interviews in epidemiological studies as in clinical studies. The classification rules and research criteria of the ICD 10 mark a definite advancement in case identification over those of the ICD 9. In my opinion, they are a good middle way between poorly defined categories and a pseudo-exactness, which moreover leads to polythetic constructs. The definition of childhood onset pervasive developmental disorder in DSM-III may serve as a negative example:

The diagnostic criteria require three obligatory symptoms and at least three out of a long list of optional symptoms. Basic data for case identification should, where possible, be collected by experts, because self-estimation and other-estimation by non-experts or parents leads to under- or overestimation of deviant behavior. The studies of Richman (1977) or Geisel et al. (1982) clearly demonstrate how parents and experts may differ in their assessment of disturbances in a child. The inexpendable use of experts stresses the importance of two-step designs even for mere economical reasons.

In particular in the context of analytical epidemiology, it seems important to diagnose concomitants of psychiatric syndromes in a narrow sense. In spite of improved diagnostical classification, case identification in specific developmental delays still raises some problems. ICD 10 roughly lists:

— specific developmental disorders of language and speech (articulation, expressive/receptive language);

— specific developmental disorders of academic skills (reading, spelling, arithmetic, mixed);

— specific developmental disorders of motor function;

— mixed specific developmental disorders.

Procedures of measurement that fit the actual concepts are not yet fully developed, though urgently called for, even for mere determination of prevalence rates. An open question in this context is, for example, how to handle the diagnosis in low IQ-ranges. In general, we proceed from a gap between nonverbal IQ and special ability as assessed on standardized tests. This difference-definition works good in the high and normal IQ-range, yet it meets with difficulties in low IQ-ranges, where we hardly find any children who fulfill the criterion (i.e., special ability two standard deviations below general intelligence).

More progress has been made in the classification of associated abnormal psychosocial situations including life events of a child. A new categorization has been developed by Rutter and the "Working-Group: Classification and Documentation of the European Society of Child and Adolescent Psychiatry," especially Poustka and Goor-Lambo (1987), to become effective with the 10th ICD revision within the wider frame of the Multiaxial Classification Scheme. Further reliability studies are yet to be expected. Poustka and Goor-Lambo propose the following classification of associated abnormal psychosocial situations:

1. abnormal intrafamilial relationships

2. familial mental disorder/deviance/handicap

3. inadequate/distorted intrafamilial communication

4. abnormal qualities of upbringing

5. abnormal immediate environment

6. acute life events

7. societal stressors

8. chronic stress associated with school/work

9. stressful events due to the child's disorder.

The definition of so-called protective influences and life conditions has not yet been satisfactorily operationalized. Before this can be undertaken, though, some questions of conceptual nature have to be solved first (as Rutter, 1985, pointed out), because it is obviously not at all sufficient to regard the protective factors as mere counterparts of adverse psychosocial influences.

From the viewpoint of case definition and case identification there are still questions left open regarding the

— determination of severity grades,

— determination of the adaptive level, respectively the impairment score,

— procedures of measuring specific developmental delays, and

— valid assessment of associated abnormal psychosocial situations.

Problems of Descriptive and Analytical Epidemiology

We have a rather sound knowledge about prevalence rates, especially in different age groups, the only fault being that unfortunately they have been mostly collected not from the same cohort, but from cross-sectional studies. Where the case identification has been based on diagnoses, the mean disturbance rate is about 12%, dependent on regional characteristics (e.g., urban vs rural); where case identification has been based

Table 1. Prevalence of child and adolescent psychiatric disorders reported in epidemiological studies (Detzner & Schmidt, 1988).

Prevalence rates*	Studies
5–10%	Jenkins et al. (1980), Kastrup (1977, 1983, Lavik (1977)
11–15%	Jenkins et al. (1980), Kastrup (1977), Rutter et al. (1975), Werner & Smith (1979), Langner et al. (1974)
16–20%	Schmidt et al. (1982), Esser & Schmidt (1985), Lavik (1977), Castell et al. (1981)
>21%	Rutter et al. (1975)

*based on diagnoses

on symptoms, the mean rate goes up to 19% (Detzner & Schmidt, 1988) (Table 1).

Prevalences of specific developmental delays are hard to determine because of the operationalization problems just mentioned; even when narrowly defined, their prevalence varies from 7 to 11% (Esser & Schmidt, 1987).

For some psychiatric syndromes we have well-based rates of prevalence and incidence, for others we do not; the latter also applies to most specific developmental disorders. This is mainly grounded in the unsatisfactory case definition. In fact, we do not know very much about the effect of differing approaches of case definition on the prevalence rates determined.

Prevalence rates seem generally to be lower in preschool age; otherwise, they show considerable stability through childhood and early adolescence. When analytical epidemiology tries to find correlations with psychiatric disturbances, the question arises as to whether boys and girls ought to be looked at separately. The relation between age and disturbancy, as well as that between abnormal psychosocial conditions and disturbancy rate, is dependent on the sex. An example for the first phenomenon is the general tendency for childhood psychiatric disorders to be more common in boys than in girls, whereas already among teens a difference between the two sexes is no longer observed. For this school-age male preponderance, usually a combination of biological and sociological explanations is given. For the later change in disfavor of the girls—or better: the leveling of difference—we have as yet no sound hypothesis. A change in classificatory conventions seems to be a probable explanation: Childhood aggressive disorder is usually subsumed under psychiatric disorders (i.e., the health department is responsible), whereas aggressive or dissocial behavior in adolescence and early adulthood is regarded as social deviance and thus a educational or social problem. A still greater difficulty is our ignorance of how this leveling comes about, and especially which boys drop out of the group of disturbed children, so that the rates equalize. It seems that there is no difference in the way in which parents respond to and deal with children of either sex—at least in the first years of life (Plomin & DeFries, 1985). According to Plomin and DeFries (1985), there is only attenuated evidence for differences in the way in which social stress and family adversity impinge on boys and girls. This applies to early childhood; for older age groups findings are contradictory. Other studies, however, found that boys are more vulnerable to various social stressors than girls. Possibly genotype-environment interactions exercise the main influence (cf., Scarr & McCartney, 1983). Clarification of this question seems most important in view of the high persistency rates of aggressive and destructive behaviors in boys.

Obviously age plays a part as a moderator variable. Family adversity is significantly more effective in childhood than in adolescence. There is no significant interaction between family adversity and sex, although sex shows a main effect in variance explanation (Blanz et al., in preparation).

That psychosocial factors play an important part in child development seems to be uncontested. In general we examine the consequences from their interindividual variance with the expected results. Transcultural studies, however, are rare. Nevertheless, they yield very interesting results. As an example I refer to the study of Yamamoto and co-workers (1987): They examined children from six countries with a 20-event, 7-point scale on the stressfulness of unpleasant experiences. They yielded a remarkable degree of agreement in the stress ratings and in the reported incidences of life events. Beyond the overall similarities, there are some fascinating variations, as shown in Table 2. This raises the question whether life events can be rated in an absolute sense or whether they have to be regarded as a relative matter depending on the social and cultural context and their overall prevalence. In a changing society we might come to a changing view of what is a life event. For example, if it becomes more and more common that parents live together without being married, then birth of an illegitimate child most probably no longer will be regarded as a risk factor. Finally, this will include to mean that primary prevention reaches its "natural" limits: If we don't know which social conditions are, from

Table 2. Incidence (%) of children's experience of stressful life events (Yamamoto et al., 1987).

Life event	Egypt	Canada	Australia	Japan
Losing parents	42.0			2.8
Going blind	39.1	2.1		
Parental fights	54.1		79.5	
Caught in thefts	33.7			2.8
Move to new school		77.0		4.8

an absolute viewpoint damaging, we consequently cannot take universal preventive measures.

In spite of its importance for the pathogenesis of psychiatric disorders, as shown by Rutter and his group (Rutter et al., 1979), the influence of "school" as a psychosocial factor has been rather neglected in analytical epidemiology—at least in the German-speaking and Romanic countries. Trying to gain an epidemiologically relevant insight into this important institution meets with resistance from two sides: the parents and the institution itself. This reservation arises partly from the need to protect personal data, which is deplorable when compared against the possible gain of knowledge.

In analogy, the legislation of data protection hinders the establishment of case registers of children and adolescents—at least in some countries. Only with the aid of such case registers would it be possible to gather a complete data set from one catchment area by bringing together data from various institutions over a longer period of time (e.g., Wing, 1977). These are basic data for investigating the natural course of different forms of disorders as well as their course under intervention, or for investigating the probability of a change-over from one diagnosis to another in differing age groups.

The isolation of other concomitant features of psychiatric diagnoses faces more difficulties. What I have in mind here, are first and foremost biological features that urgently call for their inclusion into epidemiological studies, for example, in order to search for biological "markers" for subsequent disturbances or biological correlates of distinct disorders. This seems to be of importance for pathogenetic as well as for therapy and prevention research, especially in those forms of disorders that can be understood as the comparatively uniform final stretch of primarily very different etiopathogenetic courses of disorder. The follow-up of subsamples, for example, of infantile autism, conduct disorders, or hyperkinetic syndromes, will only be possible if we form homogeneous subpopulations for these syndromes and study them in unselected samples. With respect to the biochemical structure, it may be helpful to determine the amount of cortisol in the saliva—which, however, varies with day rhythms. Structural characteristics, for example, handedness, as a "marker" of cerebral dominance, may be considered as one of these relevant biological features: A close association between left-handedness or ambidexterity and specific language disorders in boys and a significant correlation with psychiatric syndromes in the course of development have been observed.

Because of the gap between structural and biochemical features on the one side and behavior parameters on the other, the argument has been made for an inclusion of characteristics of information processing, that is, to resort to neurophysiological, psychophysiological, and neuropsychological patterns, which also focus attention on maturational aspects. Recordings of event-related potentials and electrodermal reactions have been used so far, and these methods deserve further elaboration. In this connection I refer to the studies of Ingram in general, or to the more detailed studies of Rothenberger, showing aberrant event-related potentials in anorectic girls (Rothenberger et al., 1986).

We can therefore point out short-comings of descriptive and analytical epidemiology in:

— the determination of prevalences of specific forms of disorders,

— the determination of prevalences of specific developmental delays,

— the determination of prevalences of concomitants, as for example school influences,

— the recording of biological markers and of parameters of information processing.

Special Issues Derived from Clinical Practice

Let us now turn to a third area, which also refers to questions derived from clinical practice: knowledge of pathogenesis and of the natural course of mental disorders facilitates considerations of how to make best use of the therapeutical resources at our disposal. For this, longitudinal and cohort studies are inexpendable. They show us the stability versus change of a psychiatric disorder, the probability of spontaneous remission and of development-dependent changes, and the modification of the course by therapeutical interventions. One of the most important results of child psychiatric epidemiology is the realization that emotional disturbances—in spite of their considerable duration—show a comparatively good prognosis, in any case one far better than that of dissocial disorders, which moreover have an even higher temporal persistency (e.g., Robins, 1971; Rutter, 1979; Esser et al., 1986). This certainly has consequences for the use of limited therapeutic resources. Different courses for subsamples of disorders can justify an observation of typical courses, for example, of the hyperkinetic syndrome (cf. Predergast et al., 1988), up to a critical point, where the prognosis becomes clearer, and then to decide whether it is necessary to enter into treatment. The results of our study in Mannheim, for example, indicate that severe forms of ADD with combined aggressive symptoms have a poor outcome (Schmidt & Esser, in press); this risk group deserves special attention.

Numerous interactions between pathogenetic processes show distinct influence in childhood of the developmental background. Very few models for the clarification of these processes have so far been presented. The study on the effects of life events from age 8 to 13 by a LISREL model may serve as one

Figure 1. LISREL model: family adversity, life events, and psychiatric disorder (Allehoff et al., 1988).

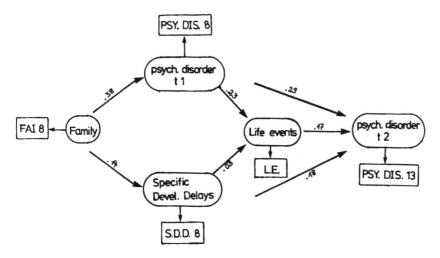

example (Allehoff et al., 1988). In general we can say the following: Life events develop their negative effects mainly in the sequel to psychiatric disorders, these in turn are triggered by chronic familial adversity (Figure 1).

For another example I refer to reflections of McGuffin and Gottesman (1985) on the possibility of determining genetically conditioned disturbances in boys and girls by means of an isocorrelational model (cf. Kidd et al., 1978; Rutter, 1970). The studies of Thomas (1987) could be mentioned here as well: He was able to prove an X-chromosomal heredity of distinctive attributes by formulating, instead of a statistical model, a mathematical model that was able to fulfill the specific conditions of the proof.

Another important methodological step are multi-generational studies. They enable us to retrace the concomitant circumstances in which nondisturbed children are raised by parents who themselves have been psychiatrically disturbed. We do have some information about hereditary risks in some disorders and about the interaction between genetic and environmental factors. Rutter's studies on "cycles of disadvantage" (Rutter & Madge, 1976) and Kolvin's study on intergenerational influences (Kolvin et al., 1983) nevertheless lead us to the assumption that intermediary factors do play an important role in determining the relations between biological and social factors. Above all, protective factors, associated abnormal psychosocial situations, and the biographical situation of the child are relevant here and demand the development of models in order to calculate the outcome and efficacy of interventions. In sum this calls for multilevel research.

Child psychiatric epidemiology must advance beyond the phase of description and work toward a formulation of models that satisfy the specific features of developmental psychopathology, that allow a comparison between normal and pathological course of development, and that can be tested for their fit.

As far as designs are concerned, the future domains of epidemiological research in child and adolescent psychiatry in my opinion are

— in the field of cohort studies,

— in the field of cross-generational studies,

— in the field of multilevel studies,

— and in the formulation of mathematical models able to describe pathogenesis and course of psychiatric disorders.

References

Achenbach, T. M. (1985). *Assessment and taxonomy of child and adolescent psychopathology.* Newbury Park, CA: Sage.

Allehoff, W. H., Esser, G., & Schmidt, M. H. (1988). Die Stellung von Life-events in kausalanalytischen Überlegungen der Kinder- und Jugendpsychiatrie: Modellbildungsversuche mit LISREL. *Zeitschrift für Kinder- und Jugendpsychiatrie, 16,* 5–13.

American Psychiatric Association (Ed.) (1980). *Diagnostic and statistical manual of mental disorders, Third edition* (DSM-III). Washington, DC: Author.

Blanz, B., Schmidt, M. H., & Esser, G. (in preparation). *The usability of the Family Adversity Index in child and adolescent psychiatric disorders.*

Detzner, M., & Schmidt, M. H. (1988). Methoden und Ergebnisse epidemiologischer Forschung. In H. Remschmidt & M. H. Schmidt (Eds.), *Kinder- und Jugendpsychiatrie in Klinik und Praxis, Vol. I* (pp. 316–333). Stuttgart: Thieme.

Esser, G., & Schmidt, M. H. (1987). *Minimale cerebrale Dysfunktion— Leerformel oder Syndrom? Empirische Untersuchung zur Bedeutung eines zentralen Konzepts in der Kinderpsychiatrie.* Stuttgart: Enke.

Esser, G., Lahnert, B., & Schmidt, M. H. (1986). Determinanten der Inanspruchnahme kinderpsychiatrisch/-psychologischer Behandlung und ihr Erfolg. *Zeitschrift für Kinder- und Jugendpsychiatrie, 14,* 228–244.

Geisel, B., Eisert, H. G., Schmidt, M. H., & Schwarzbach, H. (1982). Entwicklung und Erprobung eines Screening-Verfahrens für kinderpsychiatrisch auffällige Achtjährige (SKA 8). *Praxis der Kinderpsychologie und Kinderpsychiatrie, 31,* 173–179.

ICD 10 (1986). *International Classification of Diseases 10th Revision.* WHO Document No. 8312 Z. Geneva: World Health Organization.

Kidd, K. K., Kidd, J. R., & Records, M. A. (1978). The possible cause of the sex ratio in stuttering and its implications. *Journal of Fluency Disorder, 3,* 13–23.

Kolvin, I., Miller, F. J. W., Garside, R. F., Wolstenholme, F., & Gatzanis, S. R. M. (1983). A longitudinal study of deprivation: Life cycle changes in one generation—Implications for the next generation. In M. H. Schmidt, & H. Remschmidt (Eds.), *Epidemiological approaches in child psychiatry II* (pp. 24–42). Stuttgart: Thieme.

McGuffin, P., & Gottesman, I. I. (1985). Genetic influences on normal and abnormal development. In M. Rutter, & L. Hersov (Eds.), *Child and adolescent psychiatry—Modern approaches* (pp. 17–33). Oxford: Blackwell.

Plomin, R., & DeFries, J. C. (1985). *Origins of individual differences in infancy. The Colorado Adoption Project.* Orlando, FL: Academic Press.

Poustka, F., & Goor-Lambo, G. van (1987). *Axis Five: Associated abnormal psychosocial situations* (revised version, November, 1987). WHO document MNH/PRO/86.1. Geneva: WHO.

Predergast, M., Taylor, E., Rapoport, J. L., Bartko, J., Donnelly, M., Zametkin, A., Ahearn, M.B., Dunn, G., & Wieselberg, H. M. (1988). The diagnosis of childhood hyperactivity: A U.S.–U.K. cross-national study of DSM-III and ICD 9. *Journal of Child Psychology and Psychiatry, 29,* 289–300.

Richman, N. (1977). Is a behavior checklist for preschool children useful? In P. J. Graham (Ed.), *Epidemiological approaches in child psychiatry* (pp. 125–137). London: Academic Press.

Robins, L. N. (1971). Follow-up studies investigating childhood disorders. In E. H. Hare, & J. K. Wing (Eds.), *Psychiatric epidemiology.* London: Oxford University Press.

Rothenberger, A., Lehmkuhl, G., Kohlmeyer, K., Blanz, B., Reiser, A., & Grote, I. (1986). Anorexia nervosa (AN) in adolescents—Evoked potentials help to elucidate the biological backgrounds. In V. Gallai (Ed.), *Maturation of the CNS and evoked potentials* (pp. 375–384). Amsterdam: Elsevier.

Rutter, M. (1970). Sex differences in children's responses to family stress. In E. J. Anthony, & C. Koupernik (Eds.), *The child in his family* (pp. 165–196). New York: Wiley Interscience.

Rutter, M. (1979). *Changing youth in a changing society. Pattern of adolescent development and disorder.* London: The Nuffield Provincial Hospitals Trust.

Rutter, M. (1985). Family and school influences: Meaning, mechanisms and implications. In A. R. Nicol (Ed.), *Longitudinal studies in child psychology and psychiatry* (pp. 357–403). Chichester: John Wiley & Sons.

Rutter, M., & Madge, N. (1976). *Cycles of disadvantage.* London: Heinemann.

Rutter, M., Maughan, B., Ouston, J., & Smith, A. (1979). *Fifteen thousand hours: Secondary schools and their effects on children.* Cambridge: Harvard University Press.

Scarr, S., & McCartney, K. (1983). How people make their own environment: A theory of genotype-environment effects. *Child Development, 54,* 424–435.

Schmidt, M. H., & Esser, G. (in press). *Follow-up of young adolescents with ADD.* Paper presented at the 11th International IACAP & AP Congress, Paris 1986. To be published in *Yearbook,* Vol. 9.

Shaffer, D., Gould, M. S., Brasic, J., Ambrosini, P., Fisher, P., Bird, H., & Aluwahlia, S. (1983). A Children's Global Assessment Scale (CGAS). *Archives of General Psychiatry, 40,* 1228–1231.

Thomas, H. (1987). Modeling X-linked mediated development: development of sex differences in the service of a simple model. In J. Bisanz, C. J. Brainerd, & R. Kail (Eds.), *Formal methods of developmental psychology* (pp. 193–215). New York: Springer.

Wing, L. (1977). The use of case registers in child psychiatry and mental retardation. In P.J. Graham (Ed.), *Epidemiological approaches in child psychiatry* (pp. 31–44). London: Academic Press.

Yamamoto, K., Soliman, A., Parson, J., & Davies, O. L. (1987). Voices in unison: Stressful events in the lives of children in six countries. *Journal of Child Psychology and Psychiatry, 28,* 855–864.

Further Suggestions for Future Epidemiological Research

Frank C. Verhulst

Professor Schmidt's critique of existing knowledge gained through epidemiological methods and his suggestion for future efforts were especially aimed at three main fields of interest:

1) Assessment and taxonomy of child psychopathology;

2) methodological and analytical issues; and

3) the need for inclusion or further elaboration of psychosocial and biological parameters.

The essence of Professor Schmidt's arguments is the need for child psychiatric epidemiology to move beyond the phase of mere description and to focus on models and methods for following pathological development and for testing etiological hypotheses. In this discussion I will depart from the issues raised by Professor Schmidt and focus on some questions and suggestions that originated from our own research which is largely inspired by and partly carried out in collaboration with Professor Achenbach from the University of Vermont, U.S.A. In doing this, I realize that I can only do justice to a limited array of the suggestions Professor Schmidt has made.

The Psychometric Approach

The epidemiology of organic medical conditions ideally studies clinical disease entities that can be separated from others, have manifest or measurable etiologic agents, and show well-defined outcomes. The medical paradigm in which each syndrome is assumed to reflect a particular organic condition has been successful in identifying organic correlates of disorders such as Down syndrome and other forms of mental retardation, but has been less successful in identifying organic correlates for most psychiatric conditions in nonretarded and nonautistic children. To understand the majority of child psychiatric conditions, research may benefit from perspectives other than the medical paradigm, especially the psychometric paradigm.

Achenbach's work on standardized assessment and on empirically derived syndromes is an important exponent of this approach, which enables us to judge an individual child's score on each syndrome in relation to the scores typical of that child's sex and age (Achenbach, 1985). In this way we have an indication of the level of a child's deviance along a certain dimension. This approach may be a way to overcome an obstacle recognized by Professor Schmidt when he states that it is rather impossible to assign grades of severity of psychopathological conditions.

The psychometric approach has the advantage that qualitative as well as quantitative information can be obtained in a standardized way. However, in order to compare results from different studies, especially from studies carried out in different countries, we need to know whether standardized assessment produces similar results in different locations. Epidemiologic comparisons of behavioral/emotional problems reported for several thousand randomly selected American and Dutch children by their parents and teachers using the Achenbach CBCL revealed striking similarities (Achenbach et al., 1987a, b). Similar comparisons of results from other countries with those from the United States and Holland can even further enhance the generality of findings across different studies.

Different Informants

Obtaining information from multiple sources (e.g., parents, teachers, children, clinicians, and peers) can contribute to a comprehensive picture of a child. However, different informants having different relations to the child, and seeing the child under different conditions often disagree about the presence and severity of behavioral and emotional problems. Yet there are no systematic rules for integrating these discrepancies. Therefore, research is needed to investigate the degree and direction of discrepancies taking account of sex, age, and types of problems. We have undertaken two such studies—one in which we compared standardized ratings on behavioral/emotional problems obtained from parents and teachers (Verhulst & Akkerhuis, 1988), and one in which we compared parents' and children's reports on behavioral/emotional problems (Verhulst et al., 1987). Parents reported more problems than both children and teachers, but fears were reported more often by children, especially by the better functioning children, suggesting that children's reports of fears may be related to a higher level of adaptive functioning. Teachers scored higher on problems interfering with academic problems and on problems related to peer relations. Although we now have some "normative" data on disagreements between different informants' reports, I would like to add to Professor Schmidt's list of suggestions for future research that we need more systematic comparisons of the value of different types of data and more ways to systematically integrate information from different sources.

Summing up, I would like to add the following suggestions:

1) to carry out cross-cultural research in order to enhance the generality of findings and the possibilities for international multicenter studies;

2) to develop efficient strategies to systematically integrate information from different sources;

3) to build programmatically on replicated empirical findings.

Longitudinal Studies

Professor Schmidt has called for longitudinal studies in the field of child psychopathology. Indeed, some of the most important questions in this area concern persistence and change of children's behavioral/emotional problems and competencies across time. We recently carried out a 2-year longitudinal study of behavioral/emotional problems and competencies in a random sample from the general population of 1,412 children aged 4–14 (Verhulst & Althaus, 1988). At Time 1 parents filled in the *Child Behavior Checklist* on both occasions: at Time 1 by interview, at Time 2 by mailing and making telephone calls. The response rate was 80.2%. We analyzed the data both at interval and nominal levels. We found a significant decrease in problem scores across the two-year period, which could have been caused by the fact that at Time 2 parents were sent a questionnaire by mail, whereas the first assessment was carried out by interviews. A decrease in problem scores over time was also demonstrated, however, for clinical as well as general population samples in other studies, for instance, in the DIS study by Robins (1985). However, no satisfactory explanations are available for this phenomenon yet. It is important that studies, for instance, studies employing a retest design, take account of this phenomenon.

Irrespective of changes in the magnitude over time, stability coefficients can tell us whether individual children tend to preserve their rank orders. The stability coefficients between Time 1 and Time 2 total problem scores ranged from .62 (girls aged 4–5) to .71 (boys aged 6–11). No significant differences between stability coefficients for different age groups and for both sexes were found. This indicates that the variability of problem behavior across time in preschool children is not greater than that in older children, despite the fact that cognitive and social development show rapid changes in the preschool years; and that adolescence is not characterized by rapid changes in the levels of problems that adolescents manifest.

The highest stability was found for externalizing problems especially for the aggressive syndrome, indicating that socially less well accepted behaviors tend to persist somewhat more than problems designated as neurotic. On a categorical level, we calculated the proportion of individuals who remained disturbed across time and those individuals who improved (for details, see Verhulst & Althaus, 1988). It was found that 54% of the children from the sample who were initially classified as disturbed still scored in the disturbed range. The remaining 46% moved out of the deviant category. However, only 5% improved to a degree that placed them in the "normal" category. Our findings underscore the notion that behavioral/emotional problems should not be regarded as static. The study of child psychopathology should take account of the many variations in the types and levels of psychopathological manifestations across time. It is therefore important that changes in behavioral/emotional problems be viewed against a background of normative data.

Thus, in summing up, I come to the following suggestions:

1) More research is needed to study longitudinally the persistence and change of children's behavioral/emotional problems assessed in a standardized way.

2) Further epidemiological longitudinal research of large samples of clinically referred children is needed to clarify mechanisms involved in the persistence and change in problem behavior and competences.

References

Achenbach, T. M. (1985). Assessment and taxonomy of child and adolescent psychopathology. In A. E. Kazdin (Ed.), *Developmental clinical psychology and psychiatry.* Beverly Hills: Sage.

Achenbach, T. M., Verhulst, F. C., Baron, G. D., & Akkerhuis, G. W. (1987a). Behavioral/emotional problems and competences for ages 4 to 16. *Journal of the American Academy of Child and Adolescent Psychiatry, 26,* 317–325.

Achenbach, T. M., Verhulst, F. C., Edelbrock, C. S., Baron, G. D., & Akkerhuis, G. W. (1987b). Epidemiological comparisons of American and Dutch children: II. Behavioral/emotional problems reported by teachers for ages 6 to 11. *Journal of the American Academy of Child and Adolescent Psychiatry, 26,* 326–332.

Robins, L. N. (1985). Epidemiology: Reflections on testing the validity of psychiatric interviews. *Archive of General Psychiatry, 42,* 918–924.

Verhulst, F. C., & Althaus, M. (1988). Persistence and change in behavioral/emotional problems reported by parents of children aged 4–14: An epidemiological study. *Acta Psychiatrica Scandinavica,* Suppl. No 339, 77.

Verhulst, F. C., & Akkerhuis, G. W. (1988). Agreement between parents' and teachers' ratings of behavioral/emotional problems of children aged 4–12. *Journal of Child Psychology and Psychiatry,* in press.

Verhulst, F. C., Althaus, M., & Berden, G. F. M. G. (1987). The *Child Assessment Schedule* (CAS): Parent-child agreement and validity measures. *Journal of Child Psychology and Psychiatry, 28,* 455–466.

Indication for and Effectiveness of Specific Interventions in Child Psychiatry

Herman van Engeland

The therapeutic arsenal of child and adolescent psychiatry has expanded considerably. In addition to conventional psychodynamic approaches, usually carried out according to the child guidance model, family therapy, behavior therapy, hypnotherapy, group therapy, and pharmacotherapy have entered the field.

Recently, we had the opportunity to study the cognitive, social, and emotional functioning of children who 3–4 years before had been referred to and treated by a Regional Institute for Ambulatory Mental Health Care (Deboutte et al., 1987).

1.1% of the total population of that region was referred. About 70% of them received a regular treatment; mean duration of treatment was 12 face-to-face contacts, 30% of the treated children having more than 40 face-to-face contacts.

It turned out that three to four years later 50% of the children who had received regular treatment still scored in the clinical range on the *Child Behavior Check List* (Achenbach & Edelbrock, 1983), filled in by parents; 30% were still, or again, in treatment.

So, despite the widening of the therapeutic arsenal, the outcome of child psychiatric treatment is still a bit disappointing; research enhancing the effectiveness and efficiency of treatment is needed badly.

Clinicians are continually faced with the question: "From which theoretical perspective and by means of which interventions the disorder at hand can be treated *effectively* and *efficiently?* In order to treat a disease, syndrome, or condition, a thorough knowledge of etiology, pathogenesis, and natural course of the condition is required.

Particularly understanding the pathogenetic process is of *ultimate importance.* For example, increasing our understanding of the pathogenesis of peptic ulcer has thoroughly changed the therapeutic approach to this condition over the past two decades. Formerly rest, bedrest, distressing diets, resection of large parts of the stomach, and surgical vagotomy were considered to be rational therapeutic interventions, while leading to a decreased secretion of gastric juices. When knowledge of the mechanism underlying the secretion of gastric juices increased, the role of histamine was better understood; histamine H-2 receptor blocking agents were introduced, obviating the need for distressing diets as well as for most resections.

Our knowledge of the etiology of child psychiatric disorders has considerably expanded in the past two decades: Family disharmony, social deprivation, institutional upbringing, psychiatric disorders in one of the parents, a school environment of poor quality, cerebral lesions, and minor neurological dysfunctions have all proved to lead to an increased prevalence of child psychiatric disorders and should therefore be regarded as etiological factors. Progress has also been made in terms of our knowledge of the natural history of some conditions. The persistence of a disorder proves to be linked to the nature of that disorder (the rate of spontaneous remission in emotional disorders significantly exceeds that in conduct disorders), to the patient's sex and to persistent disharmony in the family involved.

Our understanding of the pathogenetic progress—of the way in which the presence of etiological factors in a particular individual leads to a particular, specific syndrome—lags behind and is still inadequate.

This has occurred in spite of the fact that all therapeutic techniques and interventions pretend to focus on certain pathogenetic processes. Pharmacological as well as psychological interventions are undertaken on the basis of a theory regarding the pathogenesis; all are more or less model-guided interventions. These theories, however, often have a weak empirical basis, which explains why we find it so difficult to arrive at a consensus about therapeutic strategy with regard to a particular disorder.

In my opinion consensus about therapeutic indications may be enhanced by two main research strategies!

First, an attempt should be made to consolidate the empirical basis of pathogenetic theories. A first step to achieve this lies in research into differences in the psychological, physiological, and neurochemical functioning among children suffering from different syndromes—research into *critical* psychopathological features as Ingram (this volume) has called them! Up till now, mainly *common* features, indicating psychopathology in general, were found. Most of them are described at a psychological level (certain defense mechanisms, inadequate coping mechanisms, self-image, attributional processes, etc.) and are hardly properly measurable. Up to now, the possible contribution of physiological or neurochemical variables has often remained obscure; only in the so-called neuropsychiatric syndromes like PDD and ADDH have they been studied intensively. The fact that the previously mentioned etiological factors lead more often to *internalizing* syndromes in girls and more often to *externalizing* syndromes in boys may suggest that genetic and hormonal factors, for example, by influencing hemisphere maturation, play an important role in the pathogenetic process.

The presence of *critical psychopathological features* at one of the several levels of description can support or undermine a given pathogenetic theory. The problem with research into critical features is that *homogeneous* populations must be studied, and with the available taxonomic systems, this is a difficult job, as Eric Taylor (this volume) has told us—not the least because *comorbidity factors* in children or their families burden this task considerably. Thus, this research strategy is important in order to make fundamental progress—but it is a time-consuming way we have to go!

At times we have made considerable progress in the question of rational indications without any essential improvement of our understanding of the pathogenesis of the disorder at hand. This applies for instance to *enuresis*: Comparative therapy research has given the clinician some grip. Here, behavior therapy would be the treatment of choice. Tricyclic antidepressants reduce bedwetting frequency in about 85% of the cases, but when medication stops nearly all patients relapse. In contrast, behavioral methods lead to a permanent cure in about two-thirds of cases after 2 years—provided relapses are treated in the same way. Because of their greater long-term benefits, behavioral methods are preferred to medication in the treatment of enuresis. Moreover, we can to some extent predict whether a child suffering from enuresis will or will not respond to treatment. It has been found that family disharmony is associated with a higher level of failure in the initial arrest of bedwetting and with a higher relapse rate. Behavioral deviance (as rated on a teacher questionnaire) has been found to be associated with a higher relapse rate (Shaffer, 1977). So sometimes the second research strategy, with less fundamental aims, is preferable.

Attempts should also be made to demonstrate that a given therapeutic intervention is in fact capable of producing an effect. The effects of various (alternative) interventions could be compared per syndrome, and the intervention shown to be most effective could be studied for comorbidity factors determining the child's response to therapy.

Current Situation

How much progress has been made with the two research strategies so far outlined? Without aiming at comprehensiveness, let us review the situation with regard to PDD (Pervasive Developmental Disorder), ADDH (Attention Deficit Disorder with Hyperactivity), conduct disorders, emotional disorders, and anorexia nervosa.

Much of the *PDD research* done focuses on demonstrating differences in functioning between children with a PDD syndrome and other children. At the psychological level of description, this has led to the observation that PDD children show a specific cognitive linguistic disorder and disturbed perception of social emotional information (Rutter & Schopler, 1987). Neurophysiological research into information processing has shown that children suffering from PDD have problems processing information of a higher novelty value or level of complexity (van Engeland, 1989). Biochemical research focuses on demonstrating differences in the functioning of serotonergic and dopaminergic systems in PDD children. In line with cognitive, neurophysiological, and neurochemical theories on pathogenesis, research has been done into the effects of behavioral and pharmacological therapeutic interventions respectively. Lovaas and his co-workers (1987) recently reported that intensive behavior therapy early in the course of the autistic child's life can lead to substantial improvement in cognitive functioning. This study has not yet been replicated and is regarded with some misgivings by other investigators. Even when the findings appear to be reproducible, the fact remains that the efficiency of such interventions is not very great: Forty hours of therapy per week are required over a period of several years! The effectiveness of pharmacological interventions is yet to be demonstrated convincingly (Campbell, 1988), and for differential effect studies in regard to this syndrome the time has not yet come!

Neurochemical research into the pathophysiology of *ADDH* has yielded many hypotheses but led to little factual progress (Zametkin & Rapoport, 1987). The effects of many psychotropic drugs on this syndrome have been tested, and the stimulants (methylphenidate) have thus far proved most effective. This implies that catecholamines are probably involved in some way in the pathogenesis; at least it has become clear that an effective agent should have a noradrenergic effect. Unfortunately, this noradrenergic effect, although necessary, is not *sufficient* to produce a clinical effect. Recent research has focused on determinants of the response to methylphenidate therapy: poor performance in attention tests, minor neurological dysfunctions, restlessness, and absence of emotional disorders prove to determine this response (Taylor et al., 1987).

Conduct disorders are not readily accessible to therapy. Methodologically well-designed model-guided effect studies have been sparse. Patterson and his group offer empirical evidence for the hypothesis that children with conduct disorders come from families in which coercive interaction dominates family life. On the basis of this theory, behavioral interventions (parent management) have been designed which have repeatedly shown positive effects on deviant or aggressive behavior of children both at home and in school. The child's problem behavior is normalized by these interventions, and this effect of therapy remains discernible for about one year (Kazdin, 1985). In this respect, too, something is known about the comorbidity factors that influence the response to therapy: One-parent families, maternal psychopathology, social deprivation of the family, social isolation of the family, and marital disharmony of the parents exert a negative influence on the therapeutic response. The effectiveness of parent management as well as of behavioral family therapy (Alexander et al., 1984) in conduct disorders has been convincingly demonstrated. However, it is not clear whether these therapies are more effective than other methods, because as far as I know comparative effect studies have not yet been performed.

With regard to *emotional disorders*, it may be maintained that psychotherapy, group therapy, and behavior therapy have more or less comparable effects (Hampe et al., 1971; Kolvin et al., 1981). Little is known about factors determining the therapeutic response. For the time being, it may be said that any form of psychological intervention in these disorders should be dictated solely by pragmatic and efficiency considerations. From this perspective the briefest therapy with a minimum of face-to-face encounters seems the best choice.

Family therapists have suggested that families with *anorectic* adolescents show a characteristic structure; they are believed to be "enmeshed families." Recent psychometric studies have seriously undermined this postulate (Buurmeijer & Hermans,

1988). It has been found, however, that behaviorally oriented family therapy is demonstrably effective for this syndrome, at least as far as short-term effects are concerned—a finding that still requires replication.

In view of the above, it may be maintained that the clinician aiming at short-term effects does have a few empirically documented guidelines in determining indications.

Long-Term Effects

But parents come not only for short-term effects! They also wish optimal long-term development for their child. Unfortunately, little is known about *specific* long-term effects of certain interventions. In case of ADDH it has been found that interventions with good short-term results (e.g., methylphenidate hydrochloride) do not essentially influence the long-term course of the disorder; comorbidity factors like aggressive behavior and poor peer relationships closely correlate with poor long-term outcome. Campbell and Cluss (1982) suggested that factors such as restlessness, problems in sustained attention, defective inhibitory control, and ineffective arousal regulation play an important negative role in the development of social relationships with peers. Although there are indications that methylphenidate medication causes positive changes in attentive behavior and in the social interaction between the ADDH child and his or her peers, these changes are of limited impact. Apart from the factors suggested by Campbell, there are evidently other variables that play a role in the pathogenesis of deficient social relationships with peers and in aggressive behavior.

Recent studies have disclosed some evidence in support of the hypothesis that cognitive defects and deviant social information processing play an important role in this respect (Millich & Dodge, 1984). Aggressive boys differ from boys with other psychiatric disorders and from normal boys in that they pay less attention to neutral, socially relevant information, though they do retain strongly affective positive and negative data. Aggressive boys assimilate fewer social information data before reaching a conclusion and are more likely than their non-aggressive peers to attribute hostile intent to others in ambiguous situation. When we studied the person perception of aggressive boys (Matthys et al., 1988), we found that they more frequently made statements with an extremely positive or extremely negative affective color. Further research into the determinants of and defects in social information processing seems promising and may offer new insights into the pathogenesis of persistency and chronicity.

In this field a promising treatment approach recently has developed: problem-solving skills training (PSST). This treatment focuses on cognitive processes and deficits considered to mediate maladaptive interpersonal behavior. Research has shown that child behavior at home and at school in fact can be altered by altering cognitive processing (Arbutknot & Gordon, 1986; Lochman et al., 1984). Yet most studies of PSST have focused on *non*-clinical populations and have evaluated outcomes on laboratory measures of cognitive processes. Application of these techniques to clinical populations would seem promising and therefore merits priority, at least if this can be done in the context of research into long-term effects.

Let me close with some recommendations! Progress in determining rational therapy indications can only be made by *intensifying research into the pathogenesis of disorders*. Besides that, in particular comparative research into the specific efficacy of a given intervention in a given disorder should be undertaken. In such studies outcome should be measured by multiple measurements; patients should be randomly distributed over various types of therapy; the dosage (duration and intensity) of the therapy studied should be adequate; therapies should be carried out in a standardized way (with the aid of therapy manuals!)—and preferably at several centers simultaneously!

References

Achenbach, T. M., & Edelbrock, C. (1983). *Manual for the Child Behavior Checklist and Revised Child Behavior Profile.* Burlington, VT: University of Vermont Department of Psychiatry.

Arbutknot, J., & Gordon, D. A. (1986). Behavioural and cognitive effects of a moral reasoning development intervention for high risk behaviour disordered adolescents. *Journal of Consulting Clinical Psychology, 54,* 208–216.

Buurmeijer, F. A., & Hermans, P. C. (1988). *Gezinsfunctioneren en individuele stoornissen.* Lisse: Swets and Zeitlinger.

Campbell, M. (1988). Annotation: Fenfluamine treatment in autism. *Journal of Child Psychology and Psychiatry, 29,* 1–10.

Campbell, S. D., & Cluss, P. (1982). Peer relationships of young children with behaviour problems. In K. H. Rubin, & H. S. Ross (Eds.), *Peer relationships and social skills in childhood.* New York: Springer-Verlag.

Deboutte, D., Ven, A. van de, & Engeland, H. van (1987). *Jeugd-hulpverlening geestlijke gezondheidszorg: een psychiatrisch-epide-miologische verkenning.* Rotterdam.

Engeland, H. van (1989). Psychophysiological concomitants of information processing deficits in childhood autism. In I. A. van Berck-elaer-Onnes (Ed.), *Childhood autism: diagnosis, treatment and re-search.* Lisse: Swets and Zeitlinger.

Hampe, E., Noble, H., Miller, L., & Barrett, C. (1973). Phobic children one and two years post-treatment. *Journal of Abnormal Psychology, 82,* 446–453.

Kazdin, A. (1985). *Treatment of antisocial behaviour in children and adolescents.* Homewood, IL: The Dorsey Press.

Kolvin, I., Garside, R., Nicol, A. R., Macmillan, A., Wolstenholme, F., & Leitch, I. M. (1981). *Help starts here: The maladjusted child in the ordinary school.* London: Tavistock.

Lochman, J. E., Busch, P. R., Curry, J. F., & Lapson, L. B. (1984). Treatment and generalization effects of cognitive behavioral and goal-setting interventions with aggressive boys. *Journal of Consulting and Clinical Psychology, 52,* 915–916.

Lovaas, O. I. (1987). Behavioural treatment and normal educational and intellectual functioning in young autistic children. *Journal of Consulting and Clinical Psychology, 55,* 3–9.

Matthys, W., Walterbos, W., Njio, L., & Engeland, H. van (1988). Person perception in children with conduct disorders. *Journal of Child Psychology and Psychiatry* (accepted for publication).

Millich, R., & Dodge, K. A. (1984). Social information processing in child psychiatric populations. *Journal of Abnormal Child Psychology, 12,* 471–490.

Rutter, M., & Schopler, E. (1987). Autism and pervasive developmental disorders: Concepts and diagnostic issues. *Journal of Autism and Developmental Disorders, 17,* 159–186.

Shaffer, D. (1977). Enuresis. In M. Rutter & L. Hersov (Eds.), *Child psychiatry—Modern approaches* (pp. 581–612). Oxford: Blackwell Scientific Publications.

Taylor, E., Sachar, R., Thorley, G., Wieselberg, H. M., Everitt, B., & Rutter, M. (1987). Which boys respond to stimulant medication? A controlled trial of methylphenidate in boys with disruptive behaviour. *Psychological Medicine, 17,* 121–143.

Zametkin, A. J., & Rapoport, J. L. (1987). Neurobiology of Attention Deficit Disorder with Hyperactivity: Where have we come in 50 years? *Journal of the American Academy of Child and Adolescent Psychiatry, 26,* 676–686.

Issues of Diagnosis, Intervention, and Outcome Measurement in Evaluation Research

Andreas Warnke

This topic includes the following aspects:

— *Indication of intervention:* When do we have to start what kind of therapy?

— *Effectiveness of intervention:* What has been changed toward a positive development in the patient's life and what are the secondary effects?

— *Efficacy of intervention:* How much does it cost to be effective?

Van Engeland summarized the main problems in the field of intervention research and gave recommendations for further research. We agree with his statements. A comprehensive introduction to the complex topic of intervention research in child psychiatry has been edited by Remschmidt and Schmidt (1986). Here, I would like to add some further considerations.

The evaluation of intervention methods depends on at least three variables: diagnosis, intervention methods, and measurement of intervention effectiveness and efficiency.

Diagnostic Aspects

One main statement of van Engeland is that progress in intervention research depends on a better understanding of etiology, pathogenesis, and natural course of a disorder. One aspect may be added: There is an interaction between knowledge of etiology and diagnosis, and thus treatment research also depends on the diagnostic criteria of a disorder. A good example illustrating the interaction of definitions of a syndrome and their consequences for research can be found in the appraisal of current knowledge in dyslexia, edited by Benton and Pearl (1978). Different diagnostic criteria result in inhomogeneous samples, different intervention criteria, and thus in inconsistent research data concerning effectiveness of intervention strategies.

A recommendation for future research is to promote multicenter intervention studies in which identical diagnostic and intervention criteria are used. Examples for this procedure in intervention research can be found in Remschmidt and Schmidt (1988) and Wilsher (1986).

Intervention Aspects

It is stressed by van Engeland that there is a need for comparative intervention research with a view toward the specific efficiency of different standardized intervention strategies in a given disorder. An example for this research strategy is found in the work of Sloane et al. (1975). Three aspects are offered for further consideration.

The *goals* of intervention must be clearly defined *before* the beginning of treatment, and the criteria of treatment evaluation must be directly related to these goals. Goal differences may explain inconsistencies in research results concerning short- and long-term effectiveness.

Research in *secondary effects* of psychotherapy, for example, on the control of factors of drop-out, is quite often neglected in intervention studies. Drop-out studies promise to give important information that helps to improve the compliance of the disturbed child and his or her family in intervention programs (Innerhofer & Warnke, 1978).

The *timing* of the intervention seems to be important. The syndrome itself changes according to its natural course when the patient grows older. This development of disease is well documented, for example, in the case of childhood autism (Weber, 1969). Childhood autism in baby or toddler age is associated with very different symptoms and everyday problems compared to autism in adolescence, so that very different intervention strategies are needed. The first and acute schizophrenic episode is very different from a schizophrenic defect syndrome, and in both stages of schizophrenia we have to consider very different aspects of primary, secondary, and tertiary prevention. Intervention research strategies therefore depend on homogeneous samples with respect to age of the disturbed child, his or her social situation, and the stage of the syndrome itself.

Measurement Aspects

For intervention research, van Engeland recommends recording critical features within homogeneous populations by means of a multidimensional approach, including the measurement of psychological, physiological, and neurochemical parameters. He refers as well to the fact that short-term effects are not the same as long-term effects of psychotherapy.

Two further aspects may be considered: the speed of treatment effect and the chronology of behavior change following the intervention period.

The *duration of intervention* necessary for behavior change may be an indicator of long-term effects. This fact is underlined in an evaluation study by Remschmidt and Müller (1987). Patients with anorexia nervosa who reached normal body weight within less than 47 days of inpatient treatment had a poorer prognosis compared to those anorectic patients who needed more than 47 days to attain normal weight.

Chronology of behavior change refers to the development of the manifestation of treatment effects in a follow-up period. In parent training programs for behavior management of conduct-disordered children, we had better results in the follow-up measurement 6 up to 8 months after intervention compared to results recorded in the first week after parent training (Innerhofer & Warnke, 1980).

These results support research strategies that allow a continuous measurement of intervention processes and the patient's corresponding behavior change (psychological, physiological, biochemical, social parameters) combined with follow-up studies. Follow-up studies should include, as far as possible, a complete clinical examination of the patient and should not be limited to verbal interviews or statements given in a telephone call. In parent training programs, we found impressive differences in the verbal statements of the parents and the video-controlled systematic observation data of parent-child interaction in the critical conflict situation.

Important aspects of intervention research remain undiscussed here. What we could not mention were factors of intervention settings, techniques, and different strategies of evaluation of effectiveness and efficiency. The following aspect makes clear that we need more discussion on this topic. Most children who need psychiatric help are forced to come to an institution. Many children who need help do not come. What we need is more research concerning the indication and the effectiveness of mobile outpatient intervention strategies and home treatment.

References

Benton, A. L., & Pearl, D. (Eds.) (1978). *Dyslexia. An appraisal of current knowledge.* New York: Oxford University Press.

Innerhofer, P., & Warnke, A. (1978). *Eltern als Co-Therapeuten.* Heidelberg: Springer-Verlag.

Innerhofer, P., & Warnke, A. (1980). Elterntraining nach dem Münchner Trainingsmodell. Ein Erfahrungsbericht. In H. Lukesch, M. Perrez & K. A. Schneewind (Eds.), *Familiäre Sozialisation und Intervention.* Bern: Huber.

Remschmidt, H., & Müller, H. (1987). Stationäre Gewichts-Ausgangsdaten und Langzeitprognose der Anorexia nervosa. *Zeitschrift für Kinder- und Jugendpsychiatrie, 15,* 327–341.

Remschmidt, H., & Schmidt, M. (1986). *Therapieevaluation in der Kinder- und Jugendpsychiatrie.* Stuttgart: Enke.

Remschmidt, H., & Schmidt, M. (Eds.) (1988). *Alternative Behandlungsformen in der Kinder- und Jugendpsychiatrie. Stationäre Behandlung, Tagesklinische Behandlung und Home-treatment im Vergleich.* Stuttgart: Enke.

Sloane, R. B., Staples, F. R., Cristol, A. H., Yorkston, N. J., & Whipple, K. (1975). *Psychotherapy versus behavior therapy.* Cambridge: Harvard University Press.

Weber, D. (1970). *Der frühkindliche Autismus unter dem Aspekt der Entwicklung.* Bern: Huber.

Wilsher, C. R. (1986). The nootropic concept and dyslexia. *Annals of Dyslexia, 36,* 118–137.

Play Group Therapy: Processes and Patterns and Delayed Effects

V. Bell, S. Lyne, I. Kolvin*

The crucial question about the efficacy of psychotherapy with children is now being widely addressed by careful systematic research. The doubts and uncertainties surrounding psychotherapy were thrown into sharp relief in the 1950s with Eysenck's (1952) controversial claim that adult patients receiving psychotherapy were not better off than those receiving no treatment at all. Similar claims were made in relation to psychotherapy with children (Levitt, 1957; Levitt et al., 1959). Since then, the claims and counter-claims have resounded through the therapy evaluation literature. Yet clinicians continued to practice psychotherapy, guided presumably by their own experience within the context of therapy—if not by research findings—and thereby reassured that their activities were worthwhile. The last decade has thrown up confirmatory evidence for the clinician's assumptions (Kolvin et al., 1985, 1988a, b).

Much attention is now being directed to the processes of therapy, and this paper represents an attempt to explore processes and patterns of outcome over time in relation to play group therapy. For these purposes we utilize data from previous research as outlined in *Help Starts Here* (Kolvin et al., 1985) and a more recent community-based early secondary prevention project with deprived "at risk" Inner City Children (Bell et al., 1988).

Aims

In this paper we address ourselves to four interrelated themes: *first*, the processes of therapy and their implications for outcome; *second*, the crucial importance of long-term follow-up; *third*, the importance of collecting information using multiple measures from diverse sources at different points in time; and *fourth*, the question of sleeper effects.

* I. Kolvin is indebted to the Health Promotion Trust and the Mental Health Foundation for their support.

Background

The Newcastle School-Based Study (Kolvin et al., 1985)

These studies were undertaken with 547 children identified by screening procedures; individual information was gathered from parents, teachers, and individuals by group assessments. The children were randomly allocated by school class to the various treatment regimes, including a non-treatment regime. Major follow-ups were undertaken 18 and 36 months after the baseline assessments. The treatment regime is fully described elsewhere (Kolvin et al., 1985, 1988a, b). This included behavior modifications applied in senior schools, group therapy in both primary and secondary schools, and nurture work in primary schools.

Our play groups were based on the philosophy developed by Rogers (Rogers, 1952; Hall & Lindzey, 1970). The adaptation of the group-therapy technique to younger children was influenced by the work of Axline (1947), especially her eight principles that can be followed in practical play therapy. These include the development of a warm friendly relationship with the child, accepting the child exactly as he or she is, engendering a sense of permissiveness in the relationship, being alert to the expression of feelings in the child, maintaining of a deep respect for the child's ability to solve his or her own problems, having a non-directive attitude, exerting no sense of pressure, and finally confining limitations to those that are necessary to maintain the therapy in the real world. This allows the children to reflect their feelings through play. Nevertheless, in the model established in Newcastle, it was agreed it was necessary to establish some limit setting to allow the groups to function in the complex environment of the school while at the same time strengthening internal controls of some of the more impulsive children (Axline, 1947; Ginott, 1961).

The play groups were run by trained experienced social workers who had had an additional introductory training program. They were given continuous supervision over the period of the program. The children were withdrawn from the classes for the purpose of play therapy, which was undertaken in small groups and consisted of ten sessions over one term. The groups were of mixed sex, and problems consisted of a mixture of conduct, neurotic, and educational. In the above research the processes of therapy have been described by Parker and Nicol (1981) and included monitoring of aggression, isolation, and attention-seeking behavior in any session over 17 groups.

Community-Based Early Secondary Prevention (Bell et al., 1988)

Introduction

The classical approach to prevention has been based on the work of Caplan (1964). Such phrases have been coined as "Cure is costly—prevention priceless." The most influential ideas developed in the 1960s and 1970s stated that primary preventive activities are important because they attempt to prevent the development of subsequent disorder by attacking its presumed origins, and simultaneously promote psychological adjustment (Sandford, 1965). Such primary preventive approaches do not focus directly on individual distress. In Newcastle, there has been particular interest in early secondary preventive activities, which try to identify children who are considered to be at grave risk of developing abnormally, and to prevent dysfunction from becoming severe or overt. A prominent example of early prevention were the "Head Start" programs, which were designed to facilitate educational progress by providing deprived children with compensatory stimulation. These projects were reviewed by Bronfenbrenner (1974). He concluded that compensatory stimulation provided in the preschool years gives rise to substantial IQ gains while the program lasts, but that this trend reaches a plateau and that gains are rapidly eroded once help ends. There have been some recent reviews suggesting that these programs were not without useful long-term effects.

The Newcastle research findings outlined in *Help Starts Here*, on the other hand, indicated that short-term group therapy with older children or play group therapy with younger children who were at risk for maladjustment had impressive long-term outcome. The crucial difference between the above and the "Head Start" compensatory enrichment program was that in Newcastle a therapeutic component was added. Traditionally, enrichment is geared to the cognitive and social development of the child. Play group therapy includes this but in addition it attempts to promote emotional maturational and modify any associated behavioral problems.

The *Help Starts Here* project included a number of deprived infant school children merely because maladjustment was so often inextricably interwoven with deprivation. However, the numbers of deprived children were not sufficient to enable a specific check of efficacy to be undertaken. If such efficacy can be demonstrated, then play group therapy has the potential for making a major contribution to counteracting the medium- to long-term effects of deprivation which is so widespread in our inner cities.

The Current Project

The intention of the Community-Based Secondary Prevention Project was to identify deprived infant school children and to evaluate the impact of play group therapy on them. Our hope in locating this project in the community was to make this type of prevention and intervention available in the future to a maximum number of children while causing little disruption to their lives. Inevitably, the deprived group of children included a high proportion of children who were maladjusted or at risk for maladjustment.

The project was conducted in Infant and Primary schools in an Inner City Educational Priority Area. Children in their second year at school, 5–6-year-olds, were screened using three criteria previously tested in the 1,000 Family Study (Kolvin et al., 1983, 1988a), and based on information likely to be known to the schools. These were unemployment of the breadwinner, free school meals (given to children from low-income families), and marital breakdown. During randomization, the children were matched for criteria of deprivation and sex in order to achieve a balance within the therapy groups and between these and the controls.

Each group contained 5 to 6 children, and play group therapy sessions were run over a 10-week period; these took place in schools. A total of 13 therapy groups were run. Sessions were conducted by occupational therapists, supported by a co-therapist. The previous experience of the occupational therapists included group and individual play therapy under clinical instruction and supervision. A specific training course was run for the co-therapists prior to the research project. All the therapists attended weekly supervision sessions with a psychotherapist during the course of the groups.

The assessment of the project and the collection of data has included the establishment of a baseline, followed by a short-term follow-up at 6 months after baseline, an intermediate follow-up at 12 months after baseline, and a final long-term follow-up after 24–30 months. Assessments include teacher ratings of child behavior, social and behavioral data from the parents, and assessment of verbal and reading abilities.

Again, play group therapy was modelled on principles derived from Rogers and Axline with modifications tailored to meet the needs of deprived children. We have labelled this variation "Developmental Play Group Therapy" (Jeffrey, 1984) as it attempts to meet the child's physical, emotional, and social needs as expressed through their play. It was theorized that the non-directive play setting would allow the re-experience and satisfaction of developmental needs. We used small groups of children to facilitate social learning, and provided a range of play materials for different developmental levels to facilitate growth in all areas. The therapy sessions were carried out with the consent of the parents, but their active involvement was not required. Play therapy sessions were timed to run for 45 minutes. In the non-directive play time, the therapist aimed to create a permissive and accepting environment in which the children, in the safety of a therapeutic relationship, could express themselves freely at their true level of development. Through a sensitivity to varying maturational levels, the therapist aimed, through the use of simple reflective statements, to help the children to understand themselves. This was done with individuals in the group and with the group as a whole. Social difficulties were handled in the "here and now", using clarifying statements to help the children understand their own and others' points of view. Limits were set as they were required and centered around behavior that threatened the safety and equilibrium of the group or one of its members.

Changes in Play

Previous studies have examined openness of discussion and group cohesiveness in therapy as predictors of outcome (Truax et al., 1973), but these have not been confirmed (Kolvin et al., 1985). On this occasion, we studied processes during therapy as demonstrated through play, both as a study in itself and in an attempt to define patterns of short-term changes that may be helpful as indicators of long-term outcome. The measures of play are defined in the addendum. Reliability studies have been undertaken and are reported elsewhere (Bell et al., 1988).

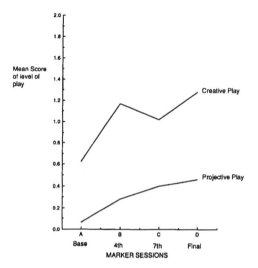

Figure 1. Changes in play (i): Increases. Play was rated on an ordinal scale (0 = none, 1 = little, 2 = some, 3 = much).

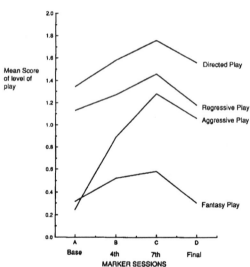

Figure 2. Changes in play (ii): Increases followed by decreases. Play was rated on an ordinal scale (0 = none, 1 = little, 2 = some, 3 = much).

The patterns are summarized in Figures 1–3. Figure 1 shows an upward trend in creative and projective play; this suggests to us a growth of self-esteem and a growth in imaginativeness. We interpret this as an improvement in the ability to use play at a more advanced level.

Figure 2 shows a pattern of increase followed by decrease; these are represented by regressive, aggressive, and fantasy forms of play. The regressive play possibly demonstrates the

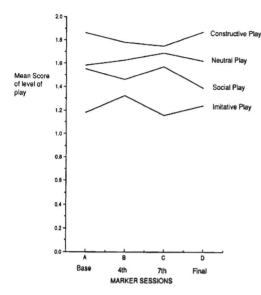

Figure 3. Changes in play (iii): Play which remains constant. Play was rated on an ordinal scale (0 = none, 1 = little, 2 = some, 3 = much).

need of some children to re-explore and transiently meet early developmental needs at the sensory/tactile and motor levels. The aggressive play perhaps indicates some of the emotional and physical tension released by these children in an environment that promotes health growth, e.g., Klein (1955), Ginott (1961), Woltmann (1955), and Salvson and Schiffer (1975). Other reasons for the rise in aggressive play were likely to be its use in challenging the boundaries of the play setting and in some cases an increased assertiveness in previously passive children.

In Figure 3 there is a representation of the type of play that remained constant. Constructive play proved to be common: It reflects the children's level of purposeful use of play materials, and we have speculated that it represents the novelty of their unrestricted availability. We would suspect that imitative and social play, which are less common but constant, will increase with the child's improved ability to socialize and to identify with the alternative adult models in their educational and play environment.

However, there are some minor fluctuations that tend to obscure major changes in a small percentage of cases. For instance, looking at the curve of social play, little change occurs, whereas looking at individuals starting with problems in cooperative play, one in four improve substantially.

In conclusion, we address ourselves to the question: Is this application of play group therapy helpful? There appear to be some immediate effects, as reflected in changes in creative and projective play and facilitatory changes as seen in aggressive and regressive play. From the monitoring of play there are indications of some short-term fluctuations occurring during therapy. While we do not rely on these as representative of improvement in itself, they may well be predictors of long-term outcome.

The Importance of Long-Term Follow-Ups

It is essential to monitor the rates of change and such changes can be compared using different formulae. First, by complex multivariate techniques such analysis of covariance (see Appendix 3 of Kolvin et al., 1985), which allow the monitoring of improvement, by which average *improvement* scores for each treatment group were compared for every measure separately at each subsequent follow-up. In addition, certain measures were summed, and the summed scored were again subject to analysis of covariance.

The second is a more simple method that calculates outcome in terms of percentages (as defined by Sainsbury, 1975, and

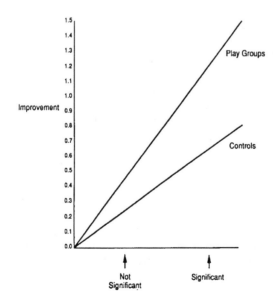

Figure 4. "Help Starts Here" (Kolvin et al., 1985): Juniors. The importance of long-term follow-up. Mean improvement in maladjustment (10 items). Here, we assume improvement is linear!

described in Appendix 2 of Kolvin et al., 1985). This allows for a calculation of the percentage who show good and moderate as opposed to poor outcome. It is noteable that the overall trends for these very different types of analyses were remarkably similar.

In their school-based intervention study, Kolvin et al. (1985) report that, over time, behavior symptoms decrease slowly but inexorably in both treated and control groups. Because of this steady reduction in symptoms in untreated disturbed children, it is unwise to assume that change constitutes improvement. It is essential that appropriate controls be selected for simultaneous study. The Newcastle research demonstrated that four-fifths of the "at-risk" children who were given play group therapy showed a good/moderate outcome as compared to just over 45% of the controls. Figure 4 demonstrates that improvement continues over time and that such improvement looks linear. However, on the basis of analysis of covariance, the differences at 18 months were not significant, though those at 36 months were highly significant.

Multiple Measures and Long-Term Follow-Up

Another crucial message from the Newcastle work is the importance of collecting information using multiple measures and from diverse sources at different points in time. It is noteable that changes occurred rather slowly, major changes appearing to occur quite a long time after therapy was complete. It seems that it is all too easy to look for the wrong things to be measured at the wrong point in time. For instance, there were some initial gains on measures of academic performance which appeared to wash out. After 18 months, there was significant improvement of only two measures (both at $p < .05$ level). In the long term, parent and teacher reports proved to be the most sensitive indicators of treatment effectiveness. Multiple measures showed significant improvement (mostly at $p < .01$ level) (Table 1). If, at the medium-term follow-up, only parent behavior scales had been employed, then the researchers could have concluded that there had been no improvement and abandoned the follow-up!

Table 1. Significant differences across time on school and home measures (paired comparisons).

Base to end of treatment	After 18 months	After 36 months
Not tested	DESB* Rutter School Scale Antisocial*	DESB** Rutter School Scale 1. Antisocial** 2. Neurotic** Newcastle Parent Scale 1. Antisocial** 2. Psychosomatic* Global measures 1. Neurotic: 5 measures* 2. Antisocial: 5 measures**

DESB = Devereux Elementary School Behaviour Rating Scale
Newcastle Parent Scale
*p < 0.05
**p < 0.01

The Question of Sleeper Effects

Despite its brevity, the effects of group therapy seem to continue for about 30 months or more, which is extraordinary in view of the many experiences the children must have had in their lives during this time. Why has this occurred? Perhaps psychotherapy merely brings forward improvement rather than actually producing change. If this were the case, we would have expected the controls to catch up. But they did not do so, and therefore we must conclude that intervention produced real change that would not otherwise have occurred. (This was not unique to our research; cf. Wright et al., 1976.) Indeed, this improvement continues and may only become evident after therapy has ceased; the mechanisms behind this are unknown, but we can advance several explanations. The first possibility is that the change is *linear*, and if we apply our measures too early, changes may be too subtle to be revealed by crude measures. Or that there is merely a non-significant trend. Unfortunately, in *Help Starts Here*, the assumed linearity may be an illusion based on the fact that we did not undertake our measures sufficiently soon after the end of treatment (Figure 5).

When we originally examined our data, we assumed that change was linear. This is a fundamental issue on both practi-

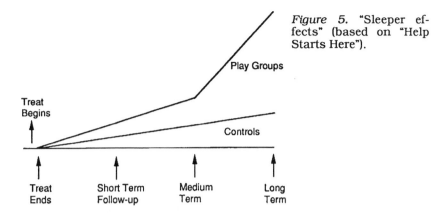

Figure 5. "Sleeper effects" (based on "Help Starts Here").

cal and theoretical grounds, and there are important questions about this. Indeed, if improvement is linear, then it should be possible to detect some trends or even significant differences at an earlier point in time. The *Help Starts Here* research (Kolvin et al., 1985) did not collect follow-up data sufficiently early to allow this question to be addressed.

In the current deprivation project using play group therapy with deprived primary school children living in our Inner City, we were able to address the question about short-term effects since we had teacher reports (Rutter B2 Scale) completed at 6 and 12 months after baseline (that is, after the initiation of the group therapy program). However, no short-term differences or even trends were identified, and under the circumstances the notion of sleeper effects begin to find favor (Figure 5).

The notion of "sleeper effects" holds considerable fascination for the therapist and researcher alike. What are sleeper phenomena—there is no problem with definition: They may be defined as delayed effects of therapy. Nor is there a problem with measuring these delayed effects. The problem for the therapist resides in understanding the *psychological processes* that precede the delayed effects, and for the researcher in how to *measure* these processes. On logical and theoretical grounds, we must assume the existence of the above psychological processes. One possibility is that over the 10 sessions of play group therapy, positive interactions between the child and peers could have resulted in greater degrees of group cohesiveness and this given rise to improvement of self-esteem, which in turn could have influenced the perceptions of that child by parents and teachers. A variation of this is that positive social interactions within the group may lead to a strengthening of relationships with peers, which may be reinforced by further contacts subsequently with these peers. These experiences may be analogous to the "fresh starts" events which George Brown considers give new perceptions to individuals who can change the course of their life. It is often noted that underlying so-called spontaneous improvement of maladjustment may be some desirable chance events that may be the turning point in an individual's life.

A second possibility is that the child may acquire a new set of skills through interactional experiences that are not useful immediately but become so at a later point in time. For instance, they may help to prepare children to cope with later stressful experiences. A third possibility is that psychotherapy affects underlying central or structural aspects of personality functioning rather than overt behavior (Wright et al., 1976). Eventually, there may be subtle shifts in personality which, through feedback mechanisms, give rise to demonstrable change in behavior, or, alternatively, that intervention has set up some latent or even subtle changes in internal psychological structures that may change the way the child perceives the environment, by changing their cognitions or attributions, and these in turn eventually give rise to a change in behavior. Thus, in the early stages there may have been changes in latent psychological structures which are only later operationalized into measurable processes.

Bearing these three possibilities in mind, tests of variation between groups may be quite irrelevant to these subtle within-subject changes. Furthermore, our data suggest that therapists should not be deterred by lack of evidence of short-term overt behavioral changes. Nevertheless, they would be wise to seek confirmation of the presence of longer-term more durable effects. Finally, if therapy has a "sleeper effect," then therapists may have to conduct therapy regardless whether it is going to have an impact.

There remain two important qualifications, and they both relate to the second treatment program. The first qualification is that we have not as yet disentangled the behavioral and environmental classifications. It is as yet not clear whether our conclusions apply to the children who are both maladjusted *and* deprived, or merely to those who are deprived but not maladjusted. The second relates to long-term follow-up. We had hoped to provide data from a final statistical analysis, but because of technical delays in analyzing data, this information is not yet available.

We do not agree with the cynic who said: "To be well adjusted is marvellous. To help others to become adjusted is even better—and less trouble."

References

Axline, V. M. (1947). *Play therapy.* Boston: Houghton Mifflin.

Bell, V., Lyne, S., & Kolvin, I. (1988). For Presentation.

Bronfenbrenner, U. (1974). *A report on longitudinal evaluation of pre-school programs.* Washington DC: US Department of Health, Education and Welfare, Office of Child Development.

Brown, G. W., & Harris, T. (1978). *Social origins of depression.* London: Tavistock.

Caplan, G. (1964). *Principles of preventive psychiatry.* London: Tavistock.

Eysenck, H. J. (1952). The effects of psychotherapy: An evaluation. *Journal of Consulting Psychology, 16,* 319–324.

Ginott, H. (1961). *Group psychotherapy with children.* New York: McGraw-Hill.

Hall, C. S., & Lindzey, G. (1970). *Theories of personality.* New York: Wiley.

Jeffrey, L. I. H. (1984). Developmental play therapy: An assessment and therapeutic technique in child psychiatry. *The British Journal of Occupational Therapy, 47,* 70–74.

Klein, M. (1955). The psychoanalytic play technique. *American Journal of Orthopsychiatry, 25,* 223–237.

Kolvin, I., Miller, F. J. W., Garside, R. F., & Gatzanis, S. R. M. (1983). One thousand families over three generations. Method and some preliminary findings. In N. Madge (Ed.), *Families at risk.* London: Heinemann.

Kolvin, I., Garside, R. F., Nicol, A. R., Macmillan, A., Wolstenholme, F., & Leitch, I. M. (1981/85). *Help Starts Here: The maladjusted child in the ordinary school.* London and New York: Tavistock Publications.

Kolvin, I., Miller, F. J. M., Fleeting, M., & Kolvin, P. A. (1988a). Social and parenting factors and offending in the Newcastle Thousand Family Study (1947–1980). *The British Journal of Psychiatry, 152,* 80–90.

Kolvin, I., Macmillan, A., Nicol, A. R., & Wrate, R. M. (1988b). Psychotherapy is effective. *Journal of the Royal Society of Medicine,* 261–266.

Levitt, E. E. (1957). The results of psychotherapy with children: An evaluation. *Journal of Consulting Psychology, 21,* 189–196.

Levitt, E. E., Beiser, H. R., & Robertson, R. E. (1959). A follow-up evaluation of cases treated at a child guidance clinic. *American Journal of Psychiatry, 29,* 337–347.

Parker, J., & Nicol, A. R. (1981). Playgroup therapy in the Junior School. II. The therapy process. *British Journal of Guidance and Counselling, 9,* 202–206.

Rogers, C. R. (1952). *Client-centred therapy.* Boston: Houghton Mifflin.

Sainsbury, P. (1975). Evaluation of community mental health programmes. In M. Guttentag & E. L. Struening (Eds.), *Handbook of evaluation research, Vol. 2* (pp. 125–160). Beverly Hills, CA: Sage.

Salvson, S. R., & Schiffer, M. (1975). *Group psychotherapies for children.* New York: International University Press.

Sandford, N. (1965). The prevention of mental illness. In B. Wolman (Ed.), *Handbook of clinical psychology* (pp. 1378–1397). New York: McGraw-Hill.

Truax, C. B., Altmann, H., Wright, L., & Mitchell, K. M. (1973). Effects of therapeutic conditions in child therapy. *Journal of Community Psychology, 1,* 313–318.

Woltmann, A. G. (1955). Concepts of play therapy techniques. *American Journal of Orthopsychiatry, 25,* 771–783.

Wright, D. M., Moelis, I., & Pollack, L. J. (1976). The outcome of individual psychotherapy: Increments at follow-up. *Journal of Child Psychology and Psychiatry, 17,* 275–285.

Appendix

Play Definitions

NEUTRAL	Play used to build a therapeutic relationship.
REGRESSIVE	The child uses play at a level below that expected for his or her chronological age and intellectual endowment, which satisfies an emotional need in the child.
AGGRESSIVE	Activity used to express aggression.
PROJECTIVE	Play used by the child to communicate feelings, fears, fantasies, etc.
FANTASY	Representational play using fantasy themes.
IMITATIVE	Representational play using themes that imitate adult activities.
SOCIAL	Cooperative play among children.
CONSTRUCTIVE	Use of toys or play materials purposefull.
CREATIVE	Child's unique influence on play materials.
DIRECTED PLAY	Structured use of the play situation by the therapist.

Methodological Problems in Investigating Long-Term Effects

Fritz Poustka

In 1973 Kolvin summarized the state of evaluation of psychiatric services for children (in England and Wales):

— there was confusion about whether the child psychiatric services were more appropriately based in health or education departments;

— planning was hampered by the lack of acceptable definitions and classifications of childhood behavior disorders;

— of those children showing psychiatric disorder in epidemiological surveys, one-third probably or definitely required treatment;

— the low percentage of parents wanting help could partly be an index of inadequate provision;

— parents' and teachers' perceptions of psychiatric disorders overlap only marginally.

Some of these statements were based on the results of the landmark in epidemiological research on child psychiatric disorders: the Isle of Wight (IOW) study (Rutter et al., 1970).

At that time Professor Kolvin's research team already started to identify by screen schoolchildren who were maladjusted or at risk for maladjustment. This was the very beginning of the "Help Starts Here" project which was designed to evaluate psychotherapeutic interventions. This project included an epidemiological design, a three-year follow-up, and a controlled evaluation of different therapeutic interventions. The results clearly demonstrate that behavioral and psychotherapeutic group interventions employed at regular schools are effective even without the parents being involved, and, what is more, that these interventions are even more effective than parent counselling or teacher consultation. Improvements not only continued long after the end of intervention, it also significantly increased the rate of spontaneous remissions from 33% to more than 50%.

Seemingly most of the questions mentioned above are solved. Is there anything left for discussion?

I want to point to problems associated with the classification and screening of psychopathology, especially regarding the problem of assessing severity and calibration of symptoms and syndromes.

From epidemiological longitudinal studies we know that chronic family discord, criminality of a parent, ineffective discipline, psychiatric disturbance of a caregiver, or other familial burden are associated with conduct disorders in children, and that parental overinvolvement is associated with emotional disorders in the children (Mattejat, 1985; Rutter, 1985). However, it is far from being clear whether and how these variables function as (causal) psychosocial risk factors in severe psychiatric conditions, e.g., obsessive-compulsive disorders, early onset psychoses, bulimic anorexia, chronic mutism, multiple tics, Asperger's syndrome, chronic school phobia, and so forth, which are much more often seen by clinicians than in epidemiological surveys.

Unlike the "Help Starts Here" project (Kolvin et al., 1981), Professor Kolvin directed his screening of children solely on such information as unemployment, low family income, marital breakdown—thus on social and familial risks and not on the child's psychopathology. There is ample evidence—again from epidemiological studies whether done in Newcastle or in Mannheim—that such adversities are good indicators for later child psychiatric disorders. But at what stage of a preventive approach are they solely sufficient to serve as the basis for screening?

Let me point to a few studies for this discussion: Unlike West's (1982) and Farrington's (1978) studies on antisocial behavior, Lee Robins (1978), in comparing four cohorts, could demonstrate that adult antisocial behavior is better predicted by childhood behavior than by family background or social class variables.

In the Mannheim epidemiological longitudinal study (Schmidt & Esser, 1984; Esser & Schmidt, 1987), severity of psychiatric disorder turned out to be the variable with the best predictive value; family adversity explained only a relatively small amount of the variance—at least in 13-year-olds it did not seem to have much impact. It does not appear as the crucial variable for predicting disorders at the age of 8 years (in contrary to special learning disabilities).

This could be demonstrated also in a child psychiatric epidemiological study of 4- to 16-year-olds in Westphalia (FRG) by Poustka et al. (1988). Table 1 displays those variables that reflect abnormal psychosocial circumstances serving as risk factors for childhood disorders, and further those individual items with the closest correlation (using multiple stepwise regression statistics) with the psychiatric symptom score. These correlations differ according to age and sex of the children and adolescents; obviously the impact of (negative) familial, other environmental, and individual variables varies with sex and developmental stage.

Using an indirect screening measure seems to bear too many uncertainties. Because of this screening procedure, at least severity of psychopathology could have been falsely estimated

Table 1. Psychosocial and individual variables with strongest correlations to psychiatric disorders according to age and sex of children. The values indicate the age- and sex-specific psychosocial or individual variable rank ordered, corresponding to the strength of the correlation with the symptom score.

Psychosocial/ Individual situation	Age/sex group					
	1	2	3	4	5	6
1: Low socioeconomic status	4	10	7		5	
2: Redundancy	1	3	2			
3: Parental discord		4		1	3	
4: Tense parental interaction	2					
5: Negative parent–child interaction			not computed			
6: Burden with problematic sibling		5	3			3
7: Illness/disability (mother)						
8: Somatic complaints (mother)		7				
9: Illness/disability (father)		8				
10: Worrying (mother)	3					
11: Worrying (father)						
12: Depression (mother)		6	4	2	4	
13: Depression (father)			5	3		
14: Risk of alcohol abuse (father)		9	6			
15: Delinquency of parents						4
16: Past familial separation (child)			1		1	1
17: Repeated admission to hospital (child)					2	
18: Single parent		2		4		
19: Other deviant parenting situation		1				2
20: Disturbed neurological function	5			5		
21: IQ ≤85		11				

Age/sex groups:
1 = male, 4–7 years
2 = male, 8–11 years
3 = male, 12–17 years
4 = female, 4–7 years
5 = female, 8–11 years
6 = female 12–17 years

in Kolvin's study. These uncertainties are probably extented by the fact that psychiatric screening as such is difficult enough: At the European Symposium on Child Psychiatric Epidemiology in Mannheim, Rutter gave a convincing example of how investigators could rank order different children in perfect accordance and yet disagree on the rating of severity of syndromes just as perfectly (Rutter, 1983). The IOW studies can be cited to exemplify calibration difficulties: Whereas in the first investigation a 6.8% overall prevalence rate of psychiatric disorders in 10–11-year-olds was reported, a second investigation (using the same instruments) yielded an almost doubled rate of 12% (Rutter et al., 1970, 1975).

What I want to say is that we should be encouraged by the huge and very successful work of Professor Kolvin to implement these therapeutic strategies in our clinical work. These interventions seem helpful at least to speed up the reduction of behavior symptoms. But in the case of a broad clinical implementation we have to

— employ a multilevel approach of classification with combined assessment of severity of symptoms/syndromes;

— try to transfer this therapeutic work to severe syndromes in a clinical sense (thus to preventive efforts that meet more difficulties).

For the latter it would be helpful to initiate multicenter studies. However, getting several clinics under one umbrella will be an even harder strain than bringing together several school classes.

References

Esser, G., & Schmidt, M. (1987). *Minimale Cerebrale Dysfunktion— Leerformel oder Syndrom?* Stuttgart: Enke.

Farrington, D. P. (1978). The family backgrounds of aggressive youths. In L.A. Hersov, & M. Berger (Eds.), *Aggression and antisocial behaviour in childhood and adolescence* (pp. 73–93). Oxford: Pergamon.

Kolvin, I. (1973). Evaluation of psychiatric services for children in England and Wales. In J. K. Wing & H. Häfner (Eds.), *Roots of evaluation* (pp. 131–162). London: Oxford University Press.

Kolvin, I. R., Garside, R. F., Nicol, A. R., Macmillan, A., Wolstenholme, F., & Leitch, I. M. (1981). *Help starts here. The maladjusted child in the ordinary school.* London: Tavistock.

Mattejat, F. (1985). *Familie und psychische Störungen.* Stuttgart: Enke.

Poustka, F., & Schmeck, K. (1988). *Aircraft noise and mental disturbances of children and adolescents—An epidemiological survey in Westphalia.* Final report for the Minister für Umwelt, Raumplanung und Landwirtschaft für das Land Nordrhein-Westfalen (unpublished).

Robins, L. N. (1978). Sturdy childhood predictors of adult antisocial behavior: replications from longitudinal studies. *Psychological Medicine, 8,* 611–622.

Rutter, M. (1983). Epidemiological-longitudinal approaches to the study of development. In M. H. Schmidt & H. Remschmidt (Eds.), *Epidemiological approaches in child psychiatry II* (pp. 2–23). Stuttgart: Thieme.

Rutter, M. (1985). Family and school influences: Meanings, mechanisms and implications. In A.R. Nicol (Ed.), *Longitudinal studies in child psychology and psychiatry* (pp. 357–403). Chichester: Wiley.

Rutter, M., Tizard, J., & Whitemore, K. (1970). *Education, health and behaviour.* London: Longman.

Rutter, M., Cox, A., Tulping, C., Berger, M., & Yule, W. (1975). Attainment and adjustment in two geographical areas. I. The prevalence of psychiatric disorder. *British Journal of Psychiatry, 126,* 493–509.

Schmidt, M. H., & Esser, G. (1984). *Kinderpsychiatrische Auffälligkeit bei Achtjährigen. Prävalenz, Risikofaktoren und Stabilität.* Unpublished manuscript for the Herrmann-Simon-Preis, Mannheim.

West, D. I. (1982). *Delinquency. Its roots, careers and prospects.* London: Heinemann.

Possible Mechanisms of Long-Term Effectiveness

A. R. Nicol, I. Kolvin, A. Macmillan, F. Wolstenholme

Levitt must take credit for drawing attention to the need for systematic evaluation of child therapies. His reviews in the 1950s and most recently in 1971 threw down a challenge to us to demonstrate that child psychotherapies were effective. This challenge has not been diminished by the fact that Levitt's reviews have been so often and so justifiably criticized. In picking over the studies Levitt included in his reviews, Wright et al. (1976) came to an extraordinary conclusion: Not only was psychotherapy effective, but the effects could only be clearly seen if long-term follow-ups were carried out. This conclusion merits examination in a little detail.

Wright et al.'s conclusion comes from the analysis of three studies. The first is that of Lehrman. This was a case control study in which the control group consisted of 110 children whose parents had withdrawn them from treatment. In other ways, care was taken to ensure that the ratings of change were carried out independently and blind. There was significant further improvement of the treatment group between close and follow-up.

The Seeman et al. (1964) study was based on children selected as disturbed on classroom measures. There was random allocation to treatment and control groups but these groups were very small, i.e., n = 6 for each group at follow-up one year after the close of therapy. Although the outcome was indistinguishable at close of treatment, at outcome there was a significant difference on a reputation test.

Heinicke (1969) compared two levels of intensity of treatment on very small groups (n = 4 in each group). Again, significant findings emerged after a time lag of one and two years.

In comparing these three limited studies with others that did not show continued improvement of treatment effects at follow-up, Wright et al. noted that an important difference was that the treatment in these studies was more *intensive*. The problem is that with such limited numbers and difficulties in the selection of control groups, can we place much weight on these studies? Whatever the answer to this question, Wright's cautious conclusion—that follow-ups are needed in any evaluation of psychotherapy—seems eminently sensible.

The more important the question, the more difficult it is to answer, and the more sparse the relevant research findings. This "inverse research law" typifies psychotherapy research. Thus, there are a lot of studies showing immediate effects on single cases with relatively minor disorders; but the more we approach genuinely handicapping disorders and look at practical ways of relieving them, the less confidently we can turn to research findings for help. However, it is important not to be too pessimistic, as there are now studies, particularly in the behavior therapy field, which have long-term follow-ups. Examples include Miller et al. (1972) on school phobia, Kirigin et al. (1975) (quoted in Ollendick, 1986) on achievement place programs—institutional treatment of delinquency by behavior modification.

The "Help Starts Here" Study

I turn now to the Newcastle study of treatment in schools that we have come to call "Help Starts Here" (Kolvin et al., 1981). It was carried out in the 1970s. A rapid presentation of the main outlines of this large-scale study is needed before we can look at the long-term findings.

The aim of the study was the prevention and treatment of maladjustment in the school environment. The study involved children of two age groups, 7-year-olds and 11-year-olds. Within each of these age groups, three treatment programs were set up, these, together with the number of subjects in each treatment group, are shown in Table 1.

The children included in the study were identified with a multiple-criterion screen that included a teacher questionnaire, sociometry, and a group reading test for the 7-year-olds, and a teacher questionnaire, self-report questionnaire, and sociom-

7-year-olds				Table 1. The
At risk controls (n=67)	Parent-teacher counselling (n=69)	Playgroups (n=74)	Nurture work (n=60)	treatment regimes.
11-year-olds				
Maladj. controls (n=92)	Parent-teacher counselling (n=83)	Senior groups (n=73)	Behaviour modification (n=74)	

Table 2. "Help Starts Here" study (7-year-olds).

Features:
1) *School screen* in primary schools for children at risk
2) *Outcome measures:* Parent and teacher reports, peer choice, educational testing
3) *Random allocation* by class
4) *Treatments* (n=60 approx. per group)
➤No treatment control
➤Parent counselling—teacher consultation
➤"Nurture work"
➤Playgroups
5) 18-month and 3-year follow-ups.

Table 3. "Help Starts Here" study (11-year-olds).

Features:
1) *School screen* for maladjusted children in secondary school
2) *Outcome measures:* Parent and teacher reports, peer choice, educational testing, anxiety scales, attitudes to school
3) *Random allocation* by class
4) *Treatments* (n=60 approx. per group)
➤No treatment control
➤Parent counselling—teacher consultation
➤Behavior modification in classroom
➤Group therapy
5) 18-month and 3-year follow-ups.

Table 4. Assessments of change.

Two types:
1) A clinical assessment of all the evidence at each stage yielding a global diagnosis and measure of severity.
2) A statistical assessment of change scores on each separate measure using multivariate analysis of covariance.
Both methods took initial severity into account, the second factor other factors as well.

etry for the 11-year-olds. Some of the features of the methodology are shown in Tables 2 and 3.

Statistical analysis is a major issue in a project of this type. In this project, two types of analysis were undertaken, as shown in Table 4, which shows the ways that change was measured, to provide, on the one hand a clinically meaningful estimate and, on the other, a more technically sophisticated measure of outcome and improvement.

Table 5. "Help Starts Here" study: Trends in results (1).

In 7-year-olds:
➤Playgroups did best
➤Parent counselling—teacher consultation did little better than controls
➤"Nurture work" came in between.
In 11-year-olds:
➤Group therapy and behavior modification both did very well
➤Parent counselling—teacher consultation did little better than controls.

Table 5. "Help Starts Here" study: Trends in results (2).

Length of follow-up:
➤Longer follow-ups showed more dramatic results (although active treatment finished).
Generalization:
➤Anxiety-type measures affected early.
➤Wide spread of measures revealed generalization—more so later.
Therapist characteristics:
➤Open, extravert therapy effective.

Tables 5 and 6 concern the outcome of the project; they are presented briefly here in a non-quantitative form. It should be noted, in addition, that the therapies seemed to have a non-specific effect. They were not disproportionately helpful with any particular type of disorder.

This equivalence of therapies has been found in a number of studies and goes against the modern dictum that our therapy should be tailored to a specified problem with a defined patient group and under known circumstances. Miller et al. (1972) compared the value of counseling and a desensitization program for school phobia: Both differed from a no-treatment control group, but there was no difference between the two treatments.

The assessment of therapists' qualities was derived from the work of Truax and Carkhuff (1967), who developed a way of rating fragments of tapes for qualities of the therapist in the therapy session. In the "Help Starts Here" study, we rated therapists not only in the therapy session, but also from our impressions arising in the context of supervision. Truax and Carkhuff identified warmth and empathy as the key therapeutic ingredients, whereas we found extraversion, openness and assertiveness to be important (Table 7).

We can speculate that the qualities of the effective therapist may be very different in the hurly-burly of the large school than in the peaceful environment of the clinic.

Table 7. Important therapist qualities.

Strong positive correlations with:
➤Extraversion
➤Assertiveness
➤Openness
Negative correlations with some *outcome measures:*
➤Empathy
➤Warmth
➤Genuineness
➤Charm
➤Good relationships
➤Neuroticism

A recent interest in the United Kingdom has been in so-called "School Differences Research." Parents have always known that there are good and bad schools, but it is only more recently that scientists have come to agree with them. Table 8 lists some of the qualities of schools that have been associated with good reading progress, low truancy rate, and better behavior.

Table 8. Therapeutic characteristics of schools (Rutter et al., 1979; Reynolds et al., 1976).

➤Teachers prepare work
➤Mark homework promptly
➤Structure
➤Praise for good work
➤Good mix of children

Table 9. "Design" of enquiry into school and therapist effects.

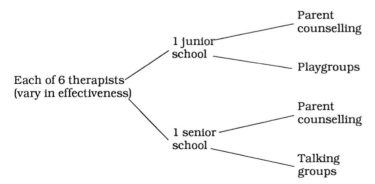

Correlate the effectiveness of therapists with different regimes and schools.

From these findings we can conclude that schools play an important part in the emotional development of children. Thus, in the "Help Starts Here" study, we can identify two possible influences in the impressive long-term effects of the treatments: therapists' effects and school effects.

At this point the discussion becomes rather tentative and is aimed at showing factors that might be taken into account in future studies rather than firm conclusions that may be derived from the present study. Table 9 outlines a "post hoc" design that attempts to disentangle the effects of school, therapist, and type of therapy. It relies on the fact that each of the six therapists worked simultaneously in a junior school and a senior school, and that they each took part in two distinct treatment programs within the two schools (one junior and one senior) within which they worked. We know that the different schools probably, and that different therapists certainly, have different levels of their therapeutic effectiveness. It may be possible in this study to differentiate the effectiveness of the six schools and of the six therapists. Table 9 shows how this might be done.

Table 10. Rank correlations of the overall change scores of six therapists in four different treatment regimes.

| | Base to midline (18 months) | | | |
	1 JPC	2 PG	3 SPC	4 SG
2	.94			
3	.89	.77*		
4	.26	.43	.43	

*Same therapist, different therapy, different school

Table 11. Rank correlations of the overall change scores of six therapists in four different treatment regimes.

| | Base to midline (3 years) | | | |
	1 JPC	2 PG	3 SPC	4 SG
2	-.14			
3	.31	-.14		
4	.09	-.20	.88*	

*Same therapist, different therapy, different school

The effectiveness of the therapists and schools are calculated by correlating the improvement scores of children who attended the same therapist giving, on the one hand, different therapies and, on the other, working in different schools. The results are presented in Table 10 for the 18-month follow-up and in Table 11 for the 3-year follow-up. A rank correlation method was used, which means that the correlations are somewhat higher than in a product moment correlation.

The most clinically important results are marked in each case with a star. In Table 10 there is a high correlation between the same therapist applying different therapy in their two different schools. This might mean that the therapist quality is important. In Table 11, the high correlation is where the school is the same but the therapy different.

These findings must be regarded as tentative, but they are consistent with the idea that the therapist is of most importance in the early stages after the therapy is given, and that at a later stage (three years) the qualities of the school environment take over as of most importance. The great importance of these findings is that they might elucidate the process by which school-based therapy has long-term beneficial effects. As psychotherapists should we continue to work in the clinic or move our base to the school? It should be remembered that the "Help Starts Here" study was concerned largely with relatively mild disorders that were identified as part of a screen in school. The findings may be quite different for a clinical group. There can be little doubt that this is an area that merits further intensive investigation.

References

Heinicke, C. M. (1969). Frequency of psychotherapeutic session as a factor affecting outcome: Analysis of clinical ratings and test results. *Journal of Abnormal Psychology, 20,* 42–98.

Kolvin, I., Garside, R. F., Nicol, A. R., Macmillan, A., Wolstenholme, F., & Leitch, I. (1981). *Help Starts Here.* London: Tavistock.

Levitt, E. E. (1971). Research on psychotherapy with children. In A. E. Bergin & S. L. Garfield (Eds.), *Handbook of psychotherapy and behavior change: An empirical analysis.* New York: Wiley.

Miller, L. C., Barrett, C. L., Hampe, E., & Noble, H. (1972). Comparison of reciprocal inhibition, psychotherapy, and waiting list control for phobic children. *Journal of Abnormal Psychology, 79,* 269–279.

Ollendick, T. H. (1986). Child and adolescent behavior therapy. In S. L. Garfield & A. E. Bergin (Eds.), *Handbook of psychotherapy and behavior change* (3rd ed.) (pp. 525–564). New York: Wiley

Reynolds, D., Jones, D., & Leger, S. (1976). Schools do make a difference. *New Society, 37*, 223–225.

Rutter, M., Maughan, B., Mortimore, P., & Ouston, J. (1979). *Fifteen thousand hours.* London: Open Books.

Seeman, J., Barry, E., & Ellinwood, C. (1964). Interpersonal assessment of play therapy outcome. *Psychotherapy: Theory, Research and Practice, 1*, 64–66.

Truax, C. B., & Carkhuff, R. R. (1967). *Toward effective counselling and psychotherapy.* Chicago: Aldine.

Wright, D. M., Moelis, I., & Pollack, L. J. (1976). The outcome of individual psychotherapy: Increments at follow-up. *Journal of Child Psychology and Psychiatry, 17*, 275–285.

The Challenge of Evaluation of Intervention

Fredrik Almqvist

Evaluation of interventions based on sound indications constitutes the basis for scientific medical practice. The relative shortage of personnel and financial resources also makes it necessary to evaluate the effectiveness of mental health services for children. Symptom relief and improvement during or immediately after treatment is the goal of every intervention in child psychiatry. The long-term effects of treatment, the topic Professor Nicol addresses in his presentation, is of special interest in child psychiatry as the discipline also strives to prevent mental illness and promote mental health later in life.

The unique research project dealing with the evaluation of therapeutic intervention in an ordinary school setting, carried out by the research team in Newcastle upon Tyne by Professor Kolvin and his co-workers (Kolvin et al., 1981), is one of the few studies in this field that has a sound design, is well controlled, and deals with a large number of cases. Professor Nicol quotes the inverse research law ("the more important the question, the more difficult it is to answer") to point out the extraordinary methodological issues that have to be taken into account when we scientifically evaluate psychotherapy. This presentation focuses on these methodological issues.

The evaluation of interventions that the clinician makes in everyday clinical child psychiatric practice can, according to Lönnqvist (1984), be described as a global evaluation of how he goals of the treatment have been attained (Figure 1). The evaluation of needs, resources, goals, intervention, and outcome happens by itself and is based on clinical experience. The evaluation and the treatment process are intertwined.

A scientific evaluation of treatment examines all the different parts of the treatment process by recording and collecting data systematically. The information is organized according to previously defined criteria on which the evaluations of the different parts of the treatment process are based (Figure 2). It is easy to see that the outcome is only one of several possible important subjects for evaluation in the treatment process. The structure of mental health care facilities, from the community level to the level of methods for single intervention, and the process of how

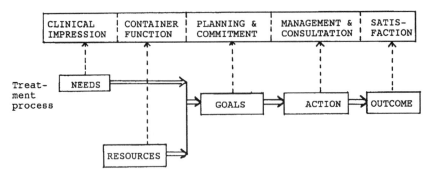

Figure 1. Global clinical evaluation of treatment (after Lönnqvist, 1984).

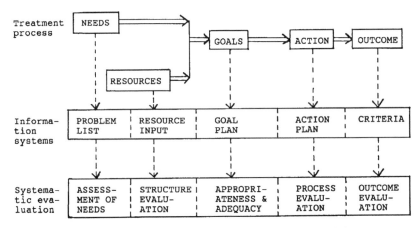

Figure 2. Systematic scientific evaluation of treatment (after Lönnqvist, 1984).

the treatment functions qualitatively and quantitatively, are two other main subjects for evaluation (Lönnqvist 1984).

Other approaches to the methodological issues are exemplified by Lee Robins (1973), who pointed to three of the most important methodological questions, namely, controlling for drop-outs, the use of different treatment methods, not only making comparisons with a no-treatment group, and finally the time for evaluation of the outcome.

Rutter's comprehensive review (1982) of the topic of psychological therapies raises three main issues, (1) the concept of disorder, (2) the therapeutic methods, and (3) the goals of treatment.

1. The theoretical preconceptions, for instance, psychoanalytical versus behavioral, influence the treatment process, the information system, and the evaluation criteria concerning such crucial issues as (a) the disorder as a function of personality imbalance or as a conditioned response, (b) symptom substitution, (c) general or specific benefit, (d) the persistence of benefit over time, (e) the significance of social and biological influence, and (f) the meaning of the child as a developing active part with a unique setting of temperament and cognition.

2. The use of specific techniques and the application of one or several therapies in one case, or the selection of methods from an arsenal of methods, is determined by theoretical orientation, personnel and financial resources, and the interests and qualities of therapists.

3. The goal of the treatment can be defined in terms of (a) symptom reduction, (b) promotion of development, (c) fostering autonomy and self-reliance, (d) generalization and persistence of improvement, and (e) changes in the environment.

Case reports and clinical series represent a descriptive design that is usually used to document clinical work. An explanatory design can be experimental or observational. In the first case, the investigator controls allocations as in clinical trials. When the investigator observes nature, he or she may, through a longitudinal design, seek causes and predictors, some of which may even be therapeutic interventions.

The Newcastle upon Tyne school project "Help Starts Here" is a very large and ambitious project in which the investigators have done almost everything possible in terms of design and methods to reach reliable results on the effectiveness of child psychiatric intervention. Through a careful selection and "matching" of the experimental groups, by applying a cross-over design with therapists and therapeutic methods, and by using a comprehensive set of methods for diagnosis and evaluation of the intervention process, the outcome and the improvement, Kolvin and his colleagues have managed to demonstrate the selective effectiveness of some therapeutic interventions and to which school, therapist, and other factors this effect relates (Kolvin et al., 1981). The long-term effects and the time-related aspects of evaluation is now highlighted in Nicol's valuable presentation.

Table 1. Methodological issues in psychiatric evaluation research.

1. Matching experimental group(s) with control groups for
   — different background factors
   — individual characteristics like psychopathology and resources
   — family attributes, with supportive or injurious effect
   — social factors like the influence of teacher and school.
2. Focusing and limiting the aims (selection)
   — severity of the disorder
   — type of disorder
3. Definition and description of the intervention(s)
   — theoretical approach
   — what kind of therapy?
   — what kind of therapist?
   — what does the therapist actually do?
   — the active ingredient of intervention.
4. Controlling confounding factors during intervention and follow-up
   — stress
   — life changes
   — school influence
   — family influence
5. Effect of treatment measured
   — during treatment
   — immediately after treatment
   — long-term effect
6. Valid and reliable methods for assessment
   — rating scales
   — structured interviews
   — bio-physiological measurments
7. Measurement of the result
   — situation-specific improvement
   — symptom-specific improvement
   — widespread effects
   — effect of normal development
8. Cost/benefit

Although this study was so well planned, with a straightforward design, it still produces complex results, basically because a great number of methods were used for measuring different aspects of treatment, especially outcome. The differences in the assessment of outcome by various methods can, however, be logically interpreted and are understandable. Another important attribute of this study is that it is so closely related to everyday life that the results are useful in clinical practice. The naturalistic feature of the design—to carry out the study in an ordinary school setting—is to some degree common to all evaluation studies of psychiatric intervention. It may be impossible to carry out a study with a design where the investigator controls allocation completely and any confounding factors have been ruled out. This is demonstrated by the variety of issues that may play a role in psychiatric evaluation studies (Table 1). We can regard a study as evaluation research when the scientific principles, methods, and theories are applied so as to make this evaluation more accurate and objective.

The Newcastle Help Starts Here project is not only one of the largest but also scientifically one of the best conducted studies in this field. The study opens a new approach in the field of child psychiatric research and especially the branch of evaluation of treatment. One may hope this study will stimulate child psychiatrists systematically to collect information about clinical activities, patients, outcome, and other characteristics of programs, personnel and products so as to improve knowledge and effectiveness, to reduce uncertainties and to make decisions about programs, methods, training and indications.

References

Kolvin,I., Garside, R.F., Nicol, A.R., Macmillan, A., Wolstenholme, F., & Leitch, I. (1981). *Help Starts Here: The maladjusted child in the ordinary school.* London: Tavistock Publications.

Lönnqvist, J. (1984) Evaluation of psychiatric treatment. *Psychiatria Fennica, 15,* 29–40.

Robins, L. N. (1973). Evaluation of psychiatric services for children. In K.J. Wing & H. Häfner (Eds.), *Roots of evaluation* (pp. 101–130). Oxford: Oxford University Press.

Rutter, M. (1982). Psychological therapies in child psychiatry: Issues and prospects. *Psycholgical Medicine, 12,* 723–740.

SECTION IV:

PERSPECTIVES OF PREVENTION RESEARCH

Conduct Problems as Predictors of Substance Abuse

Lee N. Robins*

The association between behavior problems of childhood and substance use is well established. Studies of adolescent drug users (Johnston et al., 1978; Jessor & Jessor, 1977; Kandel et al., 1978; Robins et al., 1978) have found that they have an excess of early sexual behavior, poor school performance, low aspirations for academic achievement, nonconformity with parents' rules, and that they often associate with other youngsters who are deviant in these ways. While use of psychoactive substances in childhood is not listed among the symptoms of conduct disorder in the official diagnostic nomenclature of the American Psychiatric Association, DSM-III-R (1987), it is recognized as an "associated feature," so that its presence should serve to raise the clinician's level of suspicion that the diagnosis is present, without directly contributing to the diagnosis. DSM-III-R says about children with conduct disorder: "Regular use of tobacco, liquor, or nonprescribed drugs and sexual behavior that begins unusually early for the child's peer group in his or her milieu are common."**

---

* This research was supported by the Epidemiological Catchment Area Program (ECA). The ECA is a series of five epidemiological research studies performed by independent research teams in collaboration with the staff of the Division of Biometry and Epidemiology (DBE) of the National Institute of Mental Health (NIMH). The NIMH Principal Collaborators are Darrel A. Regier, Ben Z. Locke, and Jack D. Burke, Jr.; the NIMH Project Officer is Carl A. Taube. The Principal Investigators and Co-Investigators from the five sites are Yale University, U01 MH 34224—Jerome K. Myers, Myrna M. Weissman, and Gary L. Tischler; The Johns Hopkins University U01 MH 33870—Morton Kramer and Sam Shapiro; Washington University, St. Louis, U01 MH 33883—Lee N. Robins and John E. Helzer; Duke University U01 MH 35386—Dan Blazer and Linda George; University of California, Los Angeles, U01 MH 35865—Marvin Karno, Richard L. Hough, Javier I. Escobar, M. Audrey Burnam. This work was also supported by Research Scientist Award MH 00334, USPHS Grants MH 17104, MH 31302, and DA-04001, and the MacArthur Foundation Risk Factor Network. The study reported here will be appearing also in L. N. Robins and M. L. Rutter (1989), *Straight and devious pathways to adulthood.* Cambridge: Cambridge University Press.
** We should not be misled by the fact that "begins" is a singular verb, indicating that it applies to the words closest to it—"sexual behavior"—but not to "regular use" of the listed substances. Presumably, this is a simple typographical error, because the predecessor to DSM-III-R, DSM-III (1980) says in its "Associated Features" of Conduct Disorder, "Unusually early smoking, drinking, and other substance use are also common."

To be "unusually early for his or her milieu," substance use would clearly have to occur by early adolescence in the United States. Almost all young people have had some exposure to psychoactive substances by age 18: Over 90% have had an alcoholic drink, two-thirds have smoked tobacco, and more than half have tried marijuana (Johnston et al., 1987). Smoking typically begins around age 13 or 14 (7th or 8th grade), and use of alcohol and drugs about age 15 or 16 (9th or 10th grade).

While substance *use* appears in the Associated Features for Conduct Disorder, substance *abuse,* defined as social, psychological, or physiological symptoms resulting from the use of psychoactive substances, does not. This would seem a reasonable omission, because the development of substance-abuse problems usually requires a number of years of use, by which time youngsters are past the age at which they are likely to be given a conduct disorder diagnosis (although DSM-III-R allows the diagnosis in adults, so long as it had its onset in childhood). However, occasionally problems with substances do begin in childhood or adolescence, and this fact is noted and related to conduct problems in the "Age of Onset" section of the text on Psychoactive Substance Use Disorders as follows: "Alcohol Abuse and Dependence usually appear in the 20s, 30s, and 40s. Dependence on amphetamine or similarly acting sympathomimetics, cannabis, cocaine, hallucinogens, nicotine, opioids, and phenylcyclidine (PCP) or similarly acting arylcyclohexylamines more commonly begin in the late teens or twenties.* When a psychoactive substance abuse disorder begins in early adolescence, it is often associated with conduct disorder and failure to complete school."

This statement from the Psychoactive Substance Use Disorders section linking early substance abuse with conduct disorder and the statement from the Conduct Disorder section linking conduct disorder with unusually early use of psychoactive substances may or may not imply that conduct disorder plays a causal role in either the use or abuse of substances. Neither statement specifically claims that conduct disorder determines more than the timing, i.e., the fact that use or abuse appears *early* rather than that they appear *at all.* But there are a number of hypotheses about a possible causal role for conduct disorder which are consistent with these two observations. Since it is impossible to develop problems from substances

---

* Here, another problem with number for the verb "begin"—this time its subject is "dependence," not the drugs listed; it needs an "s."

without first being exposed to them, if the early users explained by conduct disorder are an addition to the proportion of the population that would otherwise be exposed (and not just an advance in the timing of those due to use eventually), then conduct disorder is responsible for an increased rate of substance abuse by increasing the number exposed. But there are other possible pathways as well. If early use increases the risk of development of problems among those exposed, then conduct disorder contributes to substance abuse by its effect on timing alone—even if it does not increase the proportion of the population eventually exposed. A third possibility is that, in addition to its effect on timing, it has an effect on the likelihood of users' developing problems.

Exploring these three hypotheses, which are not mutually exclusive, is the goal of this chapter. We will see

— whether conduct disorder leads to more substance use over the lifetime—and thereby increases the proportion at risk of developing substance abuse;

— whether conduct disorder leads to earlier use than would otherwise occur, and whether early use itself increases the risk of developing substance abuse;

— whether conduct disorder increases the risk that use will progress into abuse, whether onset begins early or late.

Additional goals, assuming that conduct disorder is found to be a plausible contributor to the rate of substance abuse, will be to ask whether the proper definition of the causal variable is conduct disorder, considered as a diagnostic syndrome, or whether only certain of the symptoms used to make the diagnosis account for its relationship with substance use; and if the syndrome as a whole is predictive, we will ask whether the standard categorical definition of conduct disorder best explains its predictive power or whether a dimensional definition would be more useful. Finally, we will ask what conduct disorder can tell us about the repeated finding that women have less substance abuse than men. Do women have a special immunity to substance abuse beyond that provided by a lower frequency and severity of conduct disorder?

The ECA Project

The study from which our data come is the Epidemiological Catchment Area (ECA) study, conducted in five American cities during the years 1979–1985. It sampled 20,000 members of the adult population 18 years of age or older residing both in households and institutions. Respondents were interviewed three times over a 1-year period, although the middle interview asked a very limited number of questions.

Because the purpose of the study was to ascertain the prevalence of major *adult* mental disorders over the lifetime, conduct disorder was not a target diagnosis. However, antisocial personality was one of the target diagnoses, and to make that diagnosis, it was necessary to learn whether at least three childhood conduct problems had occurred before age 15. Respondents were therefore asked about each of 10 childhood behaviors, and if a behavior had occurred, they were asked the age at which it first occurred. The behaviors asked about do not cover all of the items listed as symptoms of conduct disorder in DSM-III-R. Omitted is information about forced entry into buildings, weapon use, cruelty to animals and people, and forcing sex on others. Three items are covered that are not mentioned as symptoms of conduct disorder in DSM-III-R: school discipline problems, school expulsion, and arrests. DSM-III-R items covered by our interview include lying, stealing, running away from home, fighting, truancy, and vandalism, although with respect to vandalism, we do not make the distinction between fire-setting and other destructive acts that DSM-III-R does. Thus, there is considerable overlap between conduct problems covered and the symptoms in the official nomenclature for conduct disorder, but there is not a perfect correspondence.

Among the childhood behaviors contributing to the diagnosis of antisocial personality is psychoactive substance use (alcohol or drugs) before age 15. Early substance use, as noted above, is not a symptom of conduct disorder in DSM-III-R, but only an "Associated Feature." In this chapter we will not count it as a conduct problem, but instead explore age of first use of substances as a possible consequence of conduct problems and as an independent predictor of substance abuse. We will date first substance use as the earlier of two ages—the age at first using an illicit drug and age first drunk. We asked for age first drunk rather than age at first drink because it is difficult to distinguish first self-initiated drink from sips of wine at family dinners or tastes of parents' drinks. We felt safe in assuming that getting drunk was usually self-initiated. In any case, the decision probably made little difference in the results, since Johnston et al. (1987) found that both first drink and first time drunk typically occurred in the 9th or 10th grade.

Information about conduct problems and early initiation of substance use is taken only from the first interview, since there was no opportunity for a subsequent first occurrence in a sample well over the age of 18. Problems as a result of substance use, i.e., substance abuse, reported in either the first or third interview were counted. The problems include psychological and physical dependence, social problems, withdrawal symptoms, medical problems, and emotional or mental health problems attributed to the substances. They were ascertained for each of seven categories of substances: alcohol; cannabis; cocaine; amphetamines; barbiturates; other sedatives and minor tranquilizers; hallucinogens; heroin and other opiates.

Information about childhood problems, substance use, and substance-related problems were all ascertained retrospectively. Despite our concern about the ability to recall whether these events had occurred and particularly the ages at which they had occurred, we were pleased to note that the ordering of substances used in adolescence and the relative frequency of specific conduct problems were highly consonant with results from previous surveys in which adolescents were recalling very recent events. We believe, therefore, that adults are able and willing to report reasonably accurately on behaviors in childhood and adolescence.

Results are reported for the sample weighted to compensate for design effects (e.g., interviewing only one person per household regardless of number in the household, oversampling institutional residents in all five sites, the elderly in three sites, and blacks in one site), nonresponse, and for differences between the demographic characteristics of the sampled areas and the United States as a whole. As a result, our report is our best estimate of the relationships between conduct problems and substance abuse in the United States.

Rather than reporting statistical significance of differences, which is of trivial interest in a sample so large that even a difference of one or two percent can be statistically significant, we will report relative risks and population-attributable risks—estimates of more interest for predicting the future of patients or for planning preventive programs.

Who Used Drugs

In previous analyses of these data, we found that the number of persons who had never used alcohol was small in all age and sex groups, but that there was a more sizeable minority of teetotalers in North Carolina than in the other ECA samples (Helzer & Burnham, in press). Illicit drug use was generally limited to those born after 1945, i.e., those under age 25 in 1969 when illicit drug use in the United States moved from special inner city populations into the general population (Robins et al., 1986). We also found, as have many others, that males have more use of illicit drugs than females, and that males exceed females in both alcohol and drug dependence.

Table 1 reflects these findings, when we compare the sample members who reported ever having used an illicit drug to the total sample weighted to the national population's demographic characteristics with respect to age, sex, and location.

Table 1. The sample.

	Base sample	Drug-using sample
Number	19,873	5611
	Weighted to the nation (%)	(%)
Conduct problems before age 15		
0–1	68	41
2–3	21	33
4–6	9	21
7–9	2	5
Age under 30	31	61
Age over 35	58	22
Male sex	48	56
Residence	Weighted to local populations	
New Haven	24	23
Baltimore	22	21
St. Louis	14	14
Durham	19	16
Los Angeles	21	26
Total	100	100

Drug users were overrepresented in the Los Angeles sample and underrepresented in the Durham, North Carolina, sample. Durham's lower rate is probably explained by its high rate of abstainers from alcohol, which has been called the "gateway" to illicit drugs. (Figures for the sites in Table 1 are weighted not to the nation, but to the populations resident in the areas sampled.)

Drug users were also young (61% were under 30 years of age when interviewed, and only 22% were over 35, while in the total sample, the average age was 40) and predominantly male (56%), while the total sample contained slightly more women than men, reflecting their longer life expectancy.

Drug users more often had a history of conduct disorder than did the sample as a whole. If we define conduct disorder as having had four or more conduct problems before 15, only 11% of the total population had conduct disorder, as compared with 26% of the drug users. As Figure 1 shows, the higher rate of conduct problems among males than females is what explains the predominance of males among drug users; when conduct disorders are held constant, as many women as men have used drugs. Figure 1 also clearly shows the association between youth and drug experience.

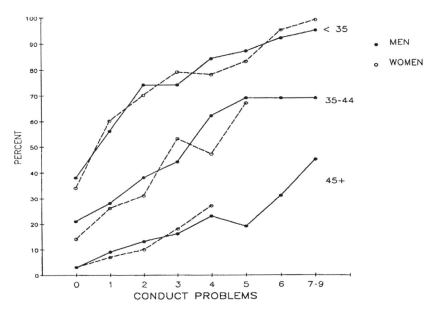

Figure 1. Drug use by age and conduct problems (for categories containing at least 20 respondents).

The high rate of conduct problems in those who have ever used illicit drugs supports our first hypothesis. One way in which conduct problems increase the risk of substance abuse is by increasing the number exposed to illicit drugs over their lifetimes. It is not just that those with conduct problems use drugs earlier than they otherwise would.

Conduct Disorder as a Predictor of Abuse by Users

We now investigate the hypotheses that conduct disorder increases the risk of substance abuse among users either by reducing the age of first exposure or by other mechanisms. To investigate these issues, we will restrict the sample to users of illicit drugs. By doing so, we assure that our sample has been exposed to both alcohol and illicit drugs, because all illicit drug users have drunk alcohol. Limiting the sample to drug users leaves us with a sample of 5,611 persons, who constitute a weighted 33% of the total sample. As noted above, this is a young, predominantly male sample.

Measuring Substance Abuse

To decide how best to reduce the description of problems with various substances to a single measure of substance abuse, we looked at responses to questions about problems with each substance in two ways: as positive diagnoses according to DSM-III criteria and as the presence of any symptom. We then did factor analyses and Guttman scale analyses, comparing results for these two definitions of abuse when substances were treated separately as listed above vs collapsing them into four categories: alcohol, cannabinoids, "pills" (sedatives, amphetamines, and hallucinogens), and "hard drugs" (cocaine and opiates). The sequence of alcohol, cannabinoids, and "other" drugs has been reported in many other studies (Kandel et al., 1978; Brunswick, 1979; O'Donnell et al., 1976). The sequence of "pills" to "hard drugs" is less well established, but worked well in the current study. Analyses were done for each of the five sample sites independently, with weighted and unweighted data. The option using four drug categories rather than seven and counting a category as positive when a problem occurred attributable to any drug in that category (rather than requiring meeting full diagnostic criteria) gave a single factor solution in every site, with high factor loadings that were almost identical whether we used weighted or unweighted data. It also produced a Guttman scale in each site, with the categories ranked from low to high as expected from previous studies: alcohol, cannabinoids, "pills," and "hard drugs," with coefficients of reproducibility all above .92 and coefficients of scalability all above .62. To choose whether to use this four category-any problem option as a Guttman scale (where a score of 0 to 4 is based on the highest level of substance with which a problem occurred) or as a simple count of the number of categories out of four in which a problem had been experienced, we correlated these two options with a number of outcomes we expected to find associated with substance abuse (e.g., job problems, arrest and illegal occupations, marital problems). Both were highly correlated with each of these outcomes, but the count of categories with at least one problem had slightly stronger correlations with these outcomes than did the Guttman scale. Therefore, in the current report, we will measure substance abuse by the number of substance categories (out of four) in which at least one problem occurred.

Table 2. Substance abuse problems among users of illicit substances.

	No. of categories with problems (5238) (%)		Substances causing problems	
None	36	1744	—	100%*
One	35	1761	*Alcohol*	69*
			Marijuana	27
			Pills	4
			Total	100
Two	18	972	*Alcohol & marijuana*	70*
			Alcohol & pills	15
			Marijuana & pills	13
			Marijuana & hard	1
			Alcohol & hard	1
			Total	100
Three	8	451	*Alcohol, mj, pills*	90*
			Mj, pills, hard	4
			Alc, mj, hard	3
			Alc, pills, hard	3
			Total	100
Four	3	260	*All four*	100*

*Sum of these categories = 83% of all users

The similarity of our count of categories with problems to a Guttman scale is shown in Table 2. When only one substance produced a problem, that substance was alcohol, as predicted by the Guttman scale, in 69% of cases. When there were problems with two substances, they were the predicted alcohol and cannabinoid in 70% of cases. When there were problems with three substances, they were the predicted alcohol, cannabinoid, and "pills" in 90% of cases. The five "ideal types" that correspond to the Guttman scale accounted for 83% of all users of illicit drugs.

Among illicit drug users, 64% developed at least one problem, but of those with a problem, most (55%) had only one, and as we noted above, this was usually with alcohol. Only 11% had problems in three or four drug categories, logically implying that they have a problem with some drug other than marijuana. Since it is drugs other than marijuana that appear to have the most serious long-term effects, we will be particularly interested in predictors of having problems with three or four categories of substances.

Demographic Predictors of Abuse among Users

Male drug users were twice as likely as female users to develop a problem, and twice as likely to have problems in three or four substances categories (Table 3). There was little difference by ethnic group in the proportion with some substance-abuse problems, though white drug users were more likely than users in other ethnic groups to have problems with three or four substances (11% vs 6% for blacks). Age groups differed little in the proportions who had experienced *any* problems with substances, but the oldest group of drug users had the lowest proportion with problems in three or four substances—even though they had had the most years since beginning use in which to develop problems.

When we look at age and sex effects simultaneously (Table 4), we find sex differences much more striking than age differences. The oldest male group (i.e., males with the lowest rate) exceeds the youngest female group (i.e., females with the highest rate) both in those who ever had a substance-abuse problem and those who had problems with three or four categories of drugs.

Table 3. Demographics of substance abuse problems among drug users.

| | | Number of categories of substances with which problems were experienced | | |
		None %	One/Two %	Three/Four %
Total		36	35	11
Sex				
	Men	24	61	14
	Women	52	41	7
Age				
	18–29	36	52	12
	30–34	38	51	11
	35+	35	57	8
Ethnic group				
	Black	39	55	6
	Hispanic	35	56	9
	White	36	53	11

Table 4. Sex and age as predictors of substance abuse problems among users.

		Men			Women		
Age	18–29	30–34	35+	18–29	30–34	35+
N	1733	613	608	1395	480	342
Categories of substance abuse	%	%	%	%	%	%
None	23	27	26	51	53	55
One or two	61	57	65	42	41	40
Three or four	16	16	9	7	6	5
Total	100	100	100	100	100	100

Conduct Problems and Substance Abuse

Syndrome or Individual Predictors

Of the nine conduct problems before age 15 about which we had information, the most frequent was truancy, occurring in three-fifths of these drug users (Table 5). Next most common was stealing, reported by more than one-third (37%). Only one in seven had been arrested, run away from home, or committed acts of vandalism before age 15.

Table 5. Individual conduct problems before age 15 as predictors of problems with three or four substances.

	Percent with this problem %	Relative risk if problem present	Population-attributable risk %
Stealing	37	3.6	49
Truancy	59	2.3	44
Expulsion/ suspension	29	3.6	43
Fighting	31	3.0	39
School discipline problem	21	3.3	32
Lying	22	2.5	25
Arrest	14	3.1	23
Vandalism	14	3.0	22
Runaway	15	2.7	21

To learn whether specific behavior predicted which users would develop substance abuse, we compared their relative risks for predicting problems in three or four categories. (The relative risk is calculated by dividing the proportion with problems in three or four categories when the conduct problem was present by the proportion with problems in that many categories when the conduct problem was absent.) Stealing and expulsion from school tied for first place, with a relative risk of 3.6. But every one of the conduct problems had a relative risk above 2.0, a common cut-off point for deciding whether a factor is "important." This narrow range means that no particular behaviors among drug users can be identified as much more predictive of substance abuse than others.

Relative risks associated with particular behaviors could be used by a clinician as a basis for predicting whether a youngster who has used drugs is at high risk of becoming a substance abuser, depending on whether or not he or she has a history of stealing, for example. But relative risks are not very useful as a basis for selecting drug users from the general population for enrollment in treatment or prevention programs. The success of such programs depends not only on whether the future course of substance abuse can be altered for the individuals selected, but also on whether the individuals who have been selected account for a high enough proportion of all probably future users so that changing their risk profile would make a major contribution to the size of the substance-abusing population. To select the proper set of individuals, it is necessary to know not only which predictors have the highest relative risks, but also how common each of these risk factors is. Changing the prospects of substance abuse only for youngsters with very rare risk factors, even if they would otherwise surely become abusers, would have little impact on the number of substance abusers in the population. A measure of risk popular with epidemiologists because it combines information about strength of the risk factor with information about its frequency is "population attributable risk" or PAR (Last, 1983). The numerator of its formula is *prevalence of the risk factor in the population* × *the relative risk − 1*; its denominator is *1 + the numerator: p(RR-1)/1+p(RR-1).*

We find that our nine conduct problems vary more in their PARs than in their relative risks, although even for the PAR, the ratio of the largest to the smallest is only slightly greater than 2 (49%/21%). Stealing has the highest PAR because it both has a high relative risk and is a common behavior problem. By identifying those who have stolen among our drug-experienced youngsters, we identify half of all who would develop serious substance abuse (according to our definition of problems in at least three categories of substances). Assuming we knew how to modify their risks, we would have to work with one-third of all drug-using children to achieve this result. Truancy has the next highest PAR, since although it has the lowest relative risk among our conduct problems, it is by far the most common of them. But if we were to use truancy as the indicator of risk, we would have to work with almost three-fifths of all drug-using children to prevent less than half of the future substance abuse. The rare behaviors—arrest, vandalism, and running away—would each require working with only one-seventh of all children, but at best would prevent less than one-fourth of all substance abuse.

If, instead of looking at individual conduct problems, we count the number present, we get a very different result (Table 6). Now we get a 27-fold difference between those who have eight or nine types of conduct problems and those who have none (55%/2%). And the risk of substance abuse rises regularly with each increase in conduct problems up to eight, indicating that for predicting substance abuse, conduct problems function well as a dimensional predictor.

When we calculate relative risks and PARs for number of conduct problems, we compare substance abuse rates in those with at least a given number of conduct problems with rates in

Table 6. Range of conduct problems before age 15 and substance abuse problems among users of drugs.

| | | Categories of substances with problems | | | |
| | | None | 1–2 | 3–4 | Total |
No. conduct problems	N	%	%	%	%
None	891	62	35	2	100
One	1015	48	49	3	100
Two	932	34	58	8	100
Three	707	27	60	13	100
Four	519	20	65	15	100
Five	426	18	61	21	100
Six	311	12	59	29	100
Seven	191	3	53	44	100
Eight	134	3	41	56	100
Nine	49	0	46	54	100

Table 7. Choosing a conduct problem cut point to predict substance abuse.

Conduct problem cut points	Proportion of drug users who would qualify (%)	Relative risk of abuse of 3–4 substances	Population attributable risk (%)
1+	81	5.9	80
2+	59	7.5	80
3+	40	5.2	63
4+	26	4.4	47
5+	17	4.6	38
6+	10	4.9	28
7+	5	5.5	18
8+	2	5.6	10
9	1	5.0	3

those with fewer conduct problems (Table 7). Every possible cut point has a higher relative risk than any individual behavior problem in Table 5, and cut points of one, two, or three have higher population-attributable risks than any of the individual problems.

Choosing a cut point requires making a compromise between the PAR, which measures the maximum possible social benefits of the intervention, assuming it was completely successful, and the cost of the intervention, as measured by the proportion of the population that would have to receive the intervention. Clearly, we would not use a cut point of one, because the PAR (benefit) is just as high with a cut point of two, while the proportion of the population receiving the intervention drops from 81% to 59%. Nor would we be likely to choose a cut point of nine because the cut point of eight provides more than three times the benefit at only twice the cost. Between two and eight, the choice would be made depending on available resources and on how effective and expensive the available interventions were believed to be.

Using a count of conduct problems is much preferable to using individual behavioral items. A cut point of four, for example, would identify about as many future substance abusers as would stealing (47% vs 49%), but would require intervening with considerably fewer drug-using youngsters (26% vs 37%). A cut point of five would identify as many prospective substance abusers as would fighting, but would require intervening with only 17% of all drug-using youngsters instead of 31%. Because number of behaviors is a more efficient predictor than type of conduct problems, our future analyses will use only number.

It is of practical utility to treat the count as a dimension rather than as a categorical value, because that allows varying the cut point with the costs and benefits of intervention. A categorical definition of conduct disorder (e.g., three or more of the listed behaviors) does not encourage this flexibility. But this advantage inheres in dimensionality only if there is no clear diagnostic threshold. If there were such a threshold, the relative risk would decline as the cut point moved above it, making the PAR drop more precipitously with increasingly restrictive cut points than it does in Table 7. The steadiness of the relative risk above the "two or more" cut point shows that there is no other diagnostic threshold for conduct problems. Thus, we conclude that for predicting substance abuse, conduct disorder can be treated as a dimensional variable within the range of two or more to eight or more conduct problems, allowing selection of cut points for intervention on the basis of resources and expected cost-benefit ratio of the selected intervention.

Age of First Use as Mechanism of Action of Conduct Disorder

Having found that conduct disorder does predict substance abuse among drug users—its impact therefore not being limited to increasing the number of users—we next want to test the hypothesis that its effect can be explained by its causing precocious use of psychoactive substances. For precocious use to

Table 8. Conduct problems and age of first substance use (mean ages).

No. of conduct problems	First time drug	First drug use	First of either
None	17.6	21.3	17.5
One	16.3	19.8	16.1
Two	15.8	18.9	15.7
Three	15.6	18.5	15.4
Four	14.7	17.8	14.4
Five	14.3	17.6	14.1
Six	14.1	16.3	13.8
Seven	12.8	16.5	12.6
Eight	12.9	16.1	12.6
Nine	12.0	14.5	12.1

Table 9. Ages of onset and number of categories of substance abuse problems.

	Age at first ...							
	Drug use				Drunkenness			
Age	<15 %	15–19 %	20–24 %	25+ %	<15 %	15–19 %	20–24 %	25+ %
No problem	13	35	45	46	16	40	55	66
One or two categories	60	53	50	51	64	51	42	34
Three or four categories	27	12	5	3	20	9	3	0
Total	100	100	100	100	100	100	100	100

be such a mechanism, conduct problems would have to predict age of first substance use, age of first substance use would have to predict substance abuse, and the effect of age of first use would have to persist when the number of conduct problems is held constant.

We found a striking relationship between number of conduct problems and early use of both drugs and alcohol (Table 8). There is more than a five-year difference in average age at first substance use between those with no conduct problems (a mean age of 17.5 years) and those with nine or more conduct problems (a mean of 12.1 years). The prediction of age at first drunkenness and age of first use of an illicit drug is equally strong. (It is noteworthy that at every level of conduct problems, first drunkenness precedes first use of illicit drugs by more than 2 years, showing the sturdiness of the alcohol use prior to drug use sequence.)

It is also the case that early drunkenness and early use of illicit drugs both predict that drug users will progress to substance abuse (Table 9). No respondent who delayed getting drunk until age 25 (or never did it) had problems in three or four categories, and two-thirds had no substance-abuse problems at all; only 3% of those who delayed illicit drug use beyond age 25 had problems with three or four categories of substances, and half had no substance-abuse problems at all. In contrast, one out of five of those who were first drunk before age 15 and one of four of those who first used a drug this young ended up with problems in three or four categories, and less than one of six escaped problems altogether.

It seems plausible, then, that conduct problems might influence later substance abuse by influencing the age at which substance use begins. The final step is to see whether age of first use continues to have a strong effect when the number of conduct problems is held constant. We find that age of onset has little or no effect if there are no conduct problems (Figure 2). Abuse is extremely rare for those free of conduct problems, no matter how early substance use began. At every other level of conduct problems, however, the earlier use begins, the greater is the likelihood of substance abuse. Thus, it is plausible that one way in which conduct problems influence substance abuse is by lowering the age of introduction to psychoactive substances.

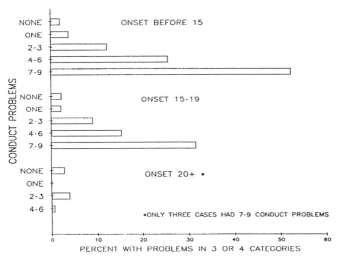

Figure 2. Conduct disorder and substance abuse, controlling on age of first use.

If this were the only mechanism through which conduct problems affected the substance abuse of users, then the relationship between conduct disorder and substance abuse would disappear when age of first use is controlled. This occurred only when substances were first used at age 20 or later. For those first using substances before age 20, number of conduct problems was an even better predictor of substance abuse than was whether use began before or after age 15. Among those beginning substance use before age 15, with seven or more conduct problems, more than half developed serious substance abuse; with only one conduct problem, only 5% did so, despite the early exposure. Indeed, for youngsters with first use before 15, the association between number of conduct problems and likelihood of serious substance abuse is as strong as for the total drug-using sample in Table 6. When first use occurred between 15 and 19 years, there is still a large effect from number of conduct problems, but the control for age of first use has somewhat reduced their impact.

These results show an interaction between conduct disorder and age of first use. Clearly, in this general population of drug users, substance abuse virtually required both having at least some early behavior problems and beginning use of substances before 20. For those first using substances earlier than that and having at least some conduct problems, the number of conduct problems did affect chances of developing substance abuse by being negatively correlated with the age of beginning use. Children with multiple conduct problems became substance abusers in part because they first used psychoactive substances before the age at which it is common "for the child's peer group in his or her milieu," but that is not the only way in which multiple conduct problems predicted substance abuse.

The results seem to convey an important message: Any delay in the introduction to alcohol or drugs appear to reduce the risk of severe substance-abuse problems, even among youngsters whose high level of conduct problems makes them especially susceptible to developing substance abuse. But a second message is that unless delay is past adolescence, youngsters with conduct disorder who use drugs will still have an elevated level of risk. We do not know what the mechanism is that links their level of conduct problems to susceptibility to substance abuse. In the absence of such understanding, preventive efforts will have to be limited to reducing use of substances, or at least attempting to postpone their use, and trying to reduce levels of conduct disorder by interventions early in childhood.

Sex Differences

Our final concern has to do with the sex of the user. We noted earlier (Table 4) that, among drug users, women were much less likely than men to develop substance-related problems. Do women have some special immunity to substance-related problems, or do they have fewer of the predictors we have already identified? In an early study (Robins et al., 1962), we found that women's apparent immunity to alcoholism was explained only by the fact that few women drink heavily; among heavy drinkers, women's rate of alcoholism as equal to that of men. This finding has been confirmed by others (Reich et al., 1975; Cloninger et al., 1978). We might expect, then, that women drug users would have fewer conduct problems than men and begin substance use later, and that if we were to control on these two predictors, that their advantage would disappear.

When we look at users of drugs (Table 10), we find that women do in fact have fewer conduct problems than men (an average of 1.8 out of 9 before age 15 vs 2.9 for men), and they do begin substance use later, first getting drunk about a year and a half later than males (at an average age of 16.6), and beginning their illicit drug use about a quarter of a year later than males (at age 19.2).

	Men	Women
Mean conduct problems before age 15 (of 9)	2.9	1.8
Mean age first drunk	15.1	16.6
Mean age first illicit drug use	18.9	19.2

Table 10. Sex differences in conduct problems and age at first substance use among users of illicit drugs.

When we look at sex differences, controlling both on age of first substance use and number of conduct problems (Figure 3), we find that women, like men, require both conduct problems and first use of substances before 20 to develop later substance abuse, and that delaying first use past age 15 does reduce risk, but that conduct problems are powerful predictors within age of first-use groups. Among those who began substance use at the "normal" time—between 15 and 18 years of age—males continue to have somewhat higher risk of substance abuse than females, even controlling on conduct problems, although differences are much less than in the total sample of users. However,

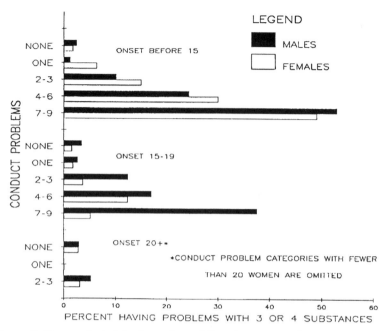

Figure 3. Comparing risks to male and female users with similar predictors.

among those who begin substance use before 15, females develop substance abuse as frequently or more frequently than males with the same level of conduct problems. These results might be explained by the fact that early use of substances is even more deviant for girls than for boys, since the "normal" age of beginning is a bit later for girls.

We have found little difference between the nature of predictors of substance abuse for male and female drug users, and we have found that the striking difference in their rates of substance abuse seems to depend on the fact that males have much more conduct disorder than females and tend to begin substance use earlier. To compare the two sexes with respect to these two predictors of substance abuse more systematically, we can use ROC curves (Erdreich & Lee, 1981; Hanley & McNeil, 1982). These curves use all possible cut-off points for number of conduct problems and age of first drug use for males and females. If conduct problems or age of first drug use was not at all predictive of substance abuse, its curve would lie on the diagonal of the square. The power of prediction of the variable is measured by the difference between the one-half of the square that lies to the right of the diagonal and the area of the square lying to the right of the ROC curves.

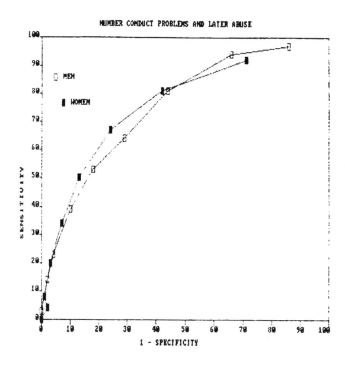

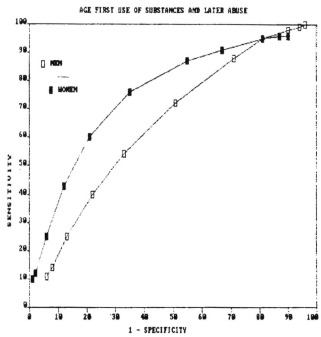

Figure 4.

For both men and women who have used drugs, conduct problems are a better predictor of later substance abuse than is age at which substance abuse began. (Compare areas below the curve in the top and bottom charts in Figure 4.) And conduct problems are equally predictive for men and women (although the best cut-off point is lower for women than men: three conduct problems vs four for men; the cut-off point nearest the upper left-hand corner is the best one). Age of first substance use is a better predictor for women than for men, as shown in the lower chart in Figure 4 (and the best cut-off point is later for women than men—below age 16 vs below age 15 for men).

Conclusions

To answer the questions we posed initially: All three of our hypotheses were supported. The connection between conduct disorder and substance abuse is partly explained by the fact that youngsters who have conduct problems are more likely than others to be exposed to illicit drugs. Among those who use illicit drugs, the more conduct problems, the earlier use begins, and early use is itself an independent predictor of abuse. But unless initial use is delayed into adulthood, the more conduct problems, the more likely is substance abuse—regardless of when use starts. Thus, conduct problems are a remarkably powerful predictor, affecting substance abuse through two identified mechanisms and independently as well.

Gender, unlike conduct problems, appears to have little direct predictive value with respect to suspectibility either to substance use or substance abuse. Although it has an indirect effect through influencing the number of conduct problems and the date at which substance use begins, girls with a history of conduct problems who start substance use early have as great a risk of later substance abuse as do boys with a similar history.

Because conduct problems continue to predict substance abuse even when we control for exposure and timing of exposure, we know those two mechanisms do not fully explain the effect of conduct problems on substance abuse. We have found that it is not the presence or absence of *particular* conduct problems that makes the difference. Further understanding of how conduct problems contribute to substance abuse will probably require information about how they influence adolescent social relationships and environments, and how they contribute to adult statuses that facilitate or inhibit heavy use of psychoactive substances. Likely adult candidates are unemployment, marital disruption, and incarceration, all known correlates of conduct disorder. Because we cannot accurately determine the temporal order of these correlates of conduct disorder relative to substance abuse in our retrospective study, we cannot test these adult outcomes as critical intervening variables between conduct disorder and substance abuse. A longitudinal research design would be particularly valuable in further explaining how conduct disorder contributes to substance abuse, as it would allow distinguishing these probably pathways of influence from the consequences of substance abuse.

We also cannot be content with our finding that one of the important mechanisms by which conduct disorder affects the risk of substance abuse is by lowering the age of first exposure to psychoactive substances. We do not yet understand why early use should be so much more dangerous than later use. It is not simply that it is an indicator of a personality profile consistent with dependence, since it is potent even for youngsters with very mild conduct problems. One wonders whether there might be a biologically critical period of high susceptibility to drug effects that ends in middle adolescence when pubertal changes are complete.

Until we have a better understanding of these age effects, and what the other intervening mechanisms are between conduct disorder and substance abuse, efforts at prevention would seem to call for reducing the number of conduct problems, avoiding the use of psychoactive substances altogether, and at least postponing their use past age 15, or better yet 19. While substance users with no history of conduct problems seem to have little risk for substance abuse even when they begin use very young, beginning use before age 15 appears to increase the risk for substance abuse among youngsters with minimal, moderate, and severe conduct problems. Even juvenile delinquents probably have a better future if they avoid early substance use and so minimize their risk of becoming abusers. Mrs. Reagan, wife of former U.S. President Ronald Reagan, instigated a campaign against drugs called "Just say 'No'." With conduct-disordered youngsters, if that fails, a campaign to "Just say 'Later'" would also seem to be useful.

References

American Psychiatric Association (1980). *Diagnostic and statistical manual of mental disorders* (3rd ed.). Washington, DC: Author.

American Psychiatric Association (1987). *Diagnostic and statistical manual of mental disorders* (3rd ed., rev.). Washington, DC: Author.

Brunswick, A. F. (1979). Black youth and drug use behavior. In G. Beschner & A. Friedman (Eds.), *Youth drug abuse: Problems, issues and treatment.* Lexington, MA: Lexington Books.

Cloninger, C. R., Christiansen, K. O., Reich, T., & Gottesman, I. I. (1978). Implications of sex differences in the prevalences of antisocial personality, alcoholism, and criminality for familial transmission. *Archives of General Psychiatry, 35,* 941–951.

Erdreich, L. S., & Lee, E. T. (1981). Use of relative operating characteristic analysis in epidemiology. *American Journal of Epidemiology, 114,* 649–662.

Hanley, J. A., & McNeil, B. J. (1982). The meaning and use of the area under a Receiver Operating Characteristic (ROC) curve. *Radiology, 143,* 29–36.

Helzer, J. E., & Burnham, A. (in press). Alcohol abuse and dependency. In L. N. Robins & D. A. Regier (Eds), *Psychiatric disorders in America.* New York: The Free Press.

Jessor, R., & Jessor, S. L. (1977). *Problem behavior and psychosocial development—A longitudinal study of youth.* New York: Academic Press.

Johnston, L., O'Malley, P., & Eveland, L. (1978). Drugs and delinquency. In D. Kandel (Ed.), *Longitudinal research on drug use: Empirical findings and methodological issues.* Washington, DC: Hemisphere-John Wiley.

Johnston, L., O'Malley, P. M., & Bachman, J. G. (1987). *National trends in drug use and related factors among American high school students and young adults.* Washington, DC: U.S. Public Health Service (DHHS Publication No. (ADM) 87-1535).

Kandel, D., Kessler, R., & Margulies, R. (1978). Adolescent initiation into stages of drug use: A developmental analysis. In D. Kandel (Ed.), *Longitudinal research on drug use: Empirical findings and methodological issues.* Washington, DC: Hemisphere-John Wiley.

Last, J. M. (1983). *A dictionary of epidemiology.* New York, Oxford, Toronto: Oxford University Press.

O'Donnell, J., Voss, H. L., Clayton, R. R., Slatin, G. T., & Room, R. G. (1976). *Young men and drugs—A nationwide survey* (Research

Monograph No. 5). Rockville, MD: National Institute on Drug Abuse.

Reich, T., Winokur, G., & Mullaney, J. (1975). The transmission of alcoholism. In R. R. Fieve, C. Rosenthal, & H. Brill (Eds.), *Genetic research in psychiatry.* Baltimore: Johns Hopkins University Press.

Robins, L. N., Bates, W. M., & O'Neal, P. (1962). Adult drinking patterns of former problem children. In D. J. Pittman & C. R. Snyder (Eds.), *Society, culture, and drinking patterns.* New York: John Wiley.

Robins, L. N., Helzer, J. E., & Przybeck. T. (1986). Substance abuse in the general population. In J. Barrett & R. M. Rose (Eds.), *Mental disorders in the community.* New York: Guilford.

Robins, L. N., Hesselbrock, M., Wish, E., & Helzer, J. E. (1978). Polydrug and alcohol use by veterans and non-veterans. In D. E. Smith, S. M. Anderson, M. Buxton, N. Gottlieb, W. Harvey, & T. Chung (Eds.), *A multicultural view of drug abuse.* Cambridge: Schenckman.

Yamaguchi, K., & Kandel, D. B. (1984). Patterns of drug use from adolescence to young adulthood: II. Sequences of progression. *American Journal of Public Health, 74,* 668–672.

Conduct Disorder and Later Substance Abuse: The Mechanisms of Continuity

Stephen Wolkind

Lee Robins' work has always been a model of what large-scale epidemiological research can offer to a medical specialty whose practitioners must focus intensely on the individual in their daily clinical practice. By looking at representative samples drawn from the general population, she provides us with a view of patterns of disturbance and relationships over time that have obvious clinical relevance. In the study presented here, she has demonstrated the—possibly not unexpected—finding that there is a powerful link between children with conduct disorders and later substance abuse or, more importantly, with problems caused by that substance abuse. Her data allow her, however, to go beyond that immediate link, and she can also demonstrate that those who have had conduct disorders began abusing psychologically active substances at an earlier age than other young people, and that this finding can in part help explain the relationship. In addition, she is able to show that, when looking at the different behavioral items constituting a conduct disorder, certain individual items have a high predictive value, but that this is of less relevance than the total number of items. There seems to be a steady additive effect, with those with a high number having a very great risk for substance abuse.

Studies such as this do have methodological problems, however. There must be reservations about the use of retrospective data and about using self-reports of current and past behavior rated—without detailed probing—during the same interview. These issues, which bedevil much developmental and psychiatric research, have been discussed in detail elsewhere (Cox & Rutter, 1985). There is need for a great deal more work on how we can best maximize the use of self-reportive and retrospective data. I think we can, however, accept Lee Robins' view that there is a face validity and an internal consistency to her findings which suggest they should be taken very seriously.

The issue that needs most consideration is what clinicians should *do* with findings such as these. Lee Robins ends her paper concentrating on the predictive efficiency of various items with the clear implication that her results should provide the basis for intervention and preventative work. Indeed, using her data, she suggests with some apparent justification, that Nancy Reagan's slogan for preventing drug abuse "Just say no" could be more realistically modified to "Just say later." Should child psychiatrists working both as clinicians and as advisors to government agencies take up this challenge and use these findings to suggest changes in drug education policy and to develop new programs to treat young people in the community who have conduct disorders? My own view is that we should be very cautious. In suggesting this I am not criticizing the quality or the results of this study; I am using Lee Robins' excellent work to comment generally on the problems of trying to translate statistical associations from epidemiological studies to preventative work in the community without understanding a great deal about the nature of the associations that have been found. The history of the dietary advice given to the general population in order to lower the prevalence of heart disease illustrates this well: Though, fortunately, a solid base for dietary education does now seem to have been reached, the early changes from sugars to fats and types of fat could well have led some to reject completely the advice being offered. With behavioral disorders, the dangers may be even greater. The classic study of McCord (1978), looking at direct intervention by social workers in the general population, is clearly very relevant here. The evidence suggests that a well-meaning program, based on apparent common sense, may have produced significant problems for those receiving the intervention, despite the fact that most of them looked back upon it in the most positive terms. More recently, Shaffer (1987) similarly reported on how a series of projects in New York designed to prevent suicide attempts by adolescents may have actually increased the rate. If we move in too quickly—and political pressures may often be very great for us to do so—we could lose all credibility, as clinicians and scientists. The importance of epidemiological findings such as those presented by Dr. Robins could then easily be discounted. The issue here is: If youngsters with conduct disorders actually delayed by a number of years the point at which they experimented with drugs, would they indeed avoid later problems with these drugs? They might—but the answer must be that we do not really know, and that they might conceivably develop even worse problems. The reason for this ignorance is that we do not yet understand the mechanisms that lie behind the association. How and in what way are conduct disorders and drugs linked?

There may not be one simple mechanism. In different subpopulations, and indeed in any one individual, there may be a number of totally different mechanisms at work. A different process might be valid for boys and girls or for members of different ethnic groups. It is essential to unravel these mechanisms and the dynamics of the links before we move on to any form of direct action that could interfere with the lives of people who have not presented themselves as patients.

The starting point should be an examination of the nature of conduct disorder itself. Classification systems such as the DSM-III-R are a way of bringing order into the chaos of communication that would otherwise exist among child psychiatrists. We should, however, be very cautious about applying a medical diagnostic system too rigidly to conduct disorders that are both medically and socially defined. The comments of Rutter (1965) on this are important. When we make a psychiatric diagnosis on a child, we are not labelling and classifying that child; what we are doing is classifying a particular type of behavior shown by that child at a particular point in time. In much longitudinal research in children (e.g., Coleman et al., 1977), the fluctuations and changes in behavior are more striking than the continuities. It becomes clear from this work that conduct disorders are not fixed categorical conditions, but rather dynamic and dimensional ones. A particular form of classificatory system may provide us with a cut-off point active at one point in time, but it does not necessarily tell us there is a specific disease that an individual either has or does not have. If we forget this, we may lose ways of thinking that could usefully explain the associations found in this study.

If we leave this idea for the moment, we can, for convenience, start with a categorical approach and look at the possible reasons for the link. Two models could be postulated, both of which might be relevant in certain circumstances. The first would imply some basic deficit in the make-up of the individual with a conduct disorder. This same deficit leads to early conduct disorder and experimentation with drugs and alcohol, which later becomes a problem. The second would suggest that both conduct disorder and drug abuse are part of the same response to an adverse or noxious influence continuously present in the environment throughout the childhood and early adulthood of the individual. The first of these suggestions has in turn a number of possibilities. One, the role of early adverse factors, either psychological or physical, occurring during the first years of life and exerting their influence over many years, has been much studied (Wolkind & Rutter, 1985). The over-whelmingly negative results suggests that for most individuals it can be virtually disregarded, though there may be some exceptions. Genetic influences could possibly be important. Though it is hard to imagine the presence of a gene or a group of genes that cause both truancy from school and a tendency to use marijuana, they might be linked by a genetically deter-mined level of impulsivity, which in turn could, of course, produce very different effects in different populations. In the present United States, it could very well greatly increase the risk for a particular individual of having both conduct and drug problems.

Behavioral genetics and neuropsychology are rapidly devel-oping fields of research. The complexity of the new work and of the technology involved is so great that child psychiatrists can no longer hope to play the amateur geneticist. They do have an essential role, however, in collaborative work in the definition and assessment of the disorders as well as the selection of the populations to be studied. The geneticist or neuropsychologist cannot play the amateur child psychiatrist. There is at present too little collaboration in these fields. Their relevance to the present study is obvious.

The apparently opposite hypothesis would move totally away from factors within the individual and focus almost wholly on the environment. It would suggest that there was a continuity in the environment, either in society in general and/or in the family, which was present throughout the childhood and early adult life of the affected individual. Thus, it might be the response of a child to a combination of poverty, poor housing, and marital disharmony between the parents that leads to a "rebellion" involving conduct problems early on and substance abuse later. The argument is that if one removes the child from this environment, the problems would cease.

The implications of these two extreme models for intervention are clearly very different. In practice, it is very likely that the link will turn out to be far more complex than either of these models and will involve a continuing dynamic interchange be-tween the individual and his or her environment. With this type of model, it is particularly important to see conduct disorder in both individual and social terms and as a dynamic, ever-chang-ing process. One could imagine how an individual, possibly vulnerable to start with, is affected by an adverse environment. This, in turn, produces a response in the individual that affects or changes that environment in a way that compounds the problem and increases the individual's chances of encountering further adverse influences. In a study of children in long-term residential care, there was a strong continuity of behavior among those originally diagnosed as having a conduct disorder. Those with this disorder, however, were far more likely than were children with emotional disorders to have been moved on to different facilities within the care system during the period of the longitudinal study (Wolkind & Renton, 1979). This lack of stability in their lives, produced at least in part by their original behavioral problems, probably contributed to the continuity.

It is worth looking briefly at the individual symptoms of conduct disorder Dr. Robins found to be most predictive. These were the child stealing and not attending school. Both these activities would, in certain environments, be very likely to bring the children into contact with individuals who are using or selling drugs. They could also lead them to be labelled as deviant and treated differently by professionals and potential employers. They could lead them to being admitted to residential facilities, where there is a culture among the young people of seeing drugs and antisocial behavior in a positive light. One could imagine a series of chain reactions beginning which bring about an accumulation of difficulties—a series of vicious cycles from which it becomes increasingly hard for the individuals to escape. Thus trapped, the children will continue to provide for themselves an environment far worse than that faced by peers.

If such a model is correct, it poses a problem for researchers in that it suggests a very fluid system in which, in theory at least, change is possible at a very large number of points in time. Random events could be of far more importance than planned interventions. Nevertheless, results such as those produced by Lee Robins do offer us real possibilities to move forward: They push us back to the concept of risk research. This type of research has fallen somewhat out of favor. Its main use in psychiatry appears to have been in the field of schizophrenia, in the attempt to identify at a very early age those individuals who would later develop the disease. The results have, on the whole, been disappointing—not surprising when we consider that even among the high-risk groups, namely, children with a schizophrenic parent, the risk is only of the order of 10%. In the field of conduct disorder and drug abuse, we are dealing with much higher probabilities. By focusing on children with differing numbers of conduct disorders who have experimented with drugs, we could produce groups with different risks of developing problems with substances as adults. The rates in any one group could range from low to very high. Relatively small groups could be followed up, the concentration being on the process by which some remain problem-free and others become trapped.

Work such as this can be time consuming and expensive, but a series of overlapping short-term individual studies would be feasible. Natural experiments such as different responses from Courts can be used to follow the process, too. Existing social welfare programs need to be evaluated carefully. It is essential that we await findings from work such as this before we jump into population intervention studies that might have no effect at all or even be detrimental. It is worth recalling the original debates about maternal deprivation. The early work in which clear associations were demonstrated between early separation and later psychopathy (Bowlby, 1946) might have suggested that widespread intervention programs be introduced to prevent early separation. With our greater understanding of the mechanisms involved in the process, we can now see how this could have been disastrous for some children. Dr. Robins' study is a first step. It provides us with many leads to follow up. It perhaps also reminds us how valuable single-case studies can be which use data that has been carefully collected by the clinician over many years.

References

Bowlby, J. (1946). *Forty four juvenile thieves.* London: Balliere, Tindall and Cox.

Coleman, J., Wolkind, S., & Ashley, J. (1977). Symptoms and behaviour disturbance and adjustment to school. *Journal of Child Psychology and Psychiatry, 18,* 201–209.

Cox, A., & Rutter, M. (1985). Diagnostic appraisal and interviewing. In M. Rutter, & L. Hersov (Eds.), *Child and adolescent psychiatry: Modern approaches* (pp. 233–248). Oxford: Blackwell.

McCord, J. (1978). A thirty year follow-up of treatment effects. *American Psychologist, 33,* 284–289.

Rutter, M. (1965). Classification and categorization in child psychiatry. *Journal of Child Psychology and Psychiatry, 6,* 71–83.

Shaffer, D. (1987). *Suicide prevention programmes for adolescents.* Paper presented to the Royal College of Psychiatrists, London.

Wolkind, S. N., & Renton, G. (1979). Psychiatric disorders in children in long term residential care: A follow-up study. *British Journal of Psychiatry, 135,* 129–135.

Wolkind, S. N., & Rutter, M. (1985). Separations, loss and family relations. In M. Rutter & L. Hersov (Eds.), *Child and adolescent psychiatry: Modern approaches* (pp. 34–57). Oxford: Blackwell.

Childhood Personality and the Prediction of Alcohol Abuse in Young Adults: A Prospective Longitudinal Study

Michael Bohman, C. Robert Cloninger, Sören Sigvardsson

Prospective longitudinal studies provide a crucial basis for evaluation of the structure and stability of personality over the life span. They also provide, inter alia, an instrument for the study of the prediction of later social adjustment, or maladjustment, which may be a prerequisite for preventive measures. There are, however, few studies that permit predictions on the relationship between childhood and adult personality. Available prospective longitudinal data have also been limited by restricted theoretical paradigms (Berger, 1982).

Most data now support an adaptive-interactive model of personality development and change, rather than fixed traits, critical stages, or learned organization (Olweus, 1980). But is difficult to quantify changes in personality because of uncertainty on how to measure the same personality construct in comparable ways at different ages. Furthermore, we cannot expect to have confident answers to questions on personality changes until we can at least specify the number of independent traits at different ages.

Factor analytic studies consistently indicate that three major dimensions of personality (in addition to intelligence) account for most observed variability in a wide variety of self-report or rater questionnaires in adults (Tellegen, 1985). These three dimensions are robust and stable across ages and cultures in both normal and abnormal samples (Cloninger, 1987; Eysenck & Long, 1986).

Studies of personality development and change in twins indicate that stable components of personality are genetically determined, and that change is largely attributable to transient environmental influences (Goldsmith, 1983). The heritabilities of personality traits are consistently estimated to lie between 40% and 60%; thus, genetic and environmental factors are roughly equally important (Loehlin, 1982). This creates an important measurement problem because pedigree studies also show that the structure of observed behavioral (i.e., phenotypic) variation does not correspond well with the structure of underlying genotypic variation. In other words, observed behavior involves the interaction of multiple genetic factors and the environment. Factors measuring observed behavior do not provide direct measures of the heritable determinants of behavior that are stable.

Recently, a theory of personality has been developed that provides an explicit and testable model of the genetically regulated dimensions underlying personality (Cloninger, 1987). This model is briefly described here in order to specify testable predictions for a prospective longitudinal study of personality from age 10 to 27 years. This study was initiated by Bohman (Bohman, 1970) in the 1960s and includes behavioral ratings on a birth cohort at ages 11, 15, 18, and 27 years. We later illustrate how this model can be used to identify antecedents of susceptibility to alcohol abuse.

A Neurobiological Model of Personality

Based on a synthesis of descriptive, genetic, neuropharmacological, and ethological data, Cloninger (1987) hypothesized that there are three dimensions of personality that are genetically independent and that have predictable patterns of interaction in their adaptive responses to novel, aversive, and appetitive stimuli. Three brain systems regulating the activation, inhibition, and maintenance of behavioral responses were hypothesized to underlie heritable individual differences in three dimensions of personality, called "novelty seeking," "harm avoidance," and "reward dependence," respectively. These dimensions and their interactions have been described in detail in adults and can be rated reliably.

Prediction of Alcohol Abuse

Several prospective longitudinal and familial high risk studies have been carried out to evaluate the possibility that premorbid personality traits are predictive of later alcoholism. Most studies have found that the premorbid traits associated with antisocial personality, including being impulsive, aggressive, overactive, distractable, impatient, and excitable are predictive of alcohol abuse in young adults. In addition, these premorbid antisocial or impulsive traits are characteristic of most early-onset alcoholics, but only a minority of alcoholics with later onset.

Late-onset alcoholism seems to be associated with passive-dependent or oral traits, such as crying easily, feeling guilty or worried, and being pessimistic, inactive, or passive.

It is obvious that alcoholism is far from being a single discrete entity. Jellinek, for instance, distinguished different subgroups of alcoholics, emphasizing the distinction between individuals who had persisting alcohol-seeking behavior ("inability to abstain entirely") and others who could abstain from alcohol for long periods but were unable to terminate drinking binges once they have started ("loss of control"). In a series of investigations (Cloninger et al., 1981; Bohman et al., 1981), we suggested two subgroups of alcoholics (Table 1).

Table 1. Distinguishing characteristics of two types of alcoholism.

Characteristic features	Type of alcoholism	
Alcohol-related problems	*Type 1*	*Type 2*
Usual age of onset (yrs)	>25	<25
Spontaneous alcohol seeking (inability to abstain)	infrequent	frequent
Fighting and arrests when drinking	infrequent	frequent
Psychological dependence (loss of control)	frequent	infrequent
Guilt and fear about alcohol dependence	frequent	infrequent
Personality traits		
Novelty seeking	low	high
Harm avoidance	high	low
Reward dependence	high	low

Type 1 alcoholism, the most common variety, is associated with loss of control, guilt, and fear about dependence on alcohol with onset developing after heavy drinking that is reinforced by external circumstances, usually in late adulthood (e.g., drinking at lunch or after work at the encouragements of friends). Loss of control and craving for alcohol appear to depend on conditioned expectancies about alcohol's effects. In contrast, *type 2 alcoholism* is associated with frequent impulsive-aggressive behavior, such as fighting or reckless driving after drinking. It is essential to note that these two groups of alcoholics have opposite extremes of bipolar personality traits that vary continuously. The development of loss of control is associated with passive-dependent or oral personalities, i.e., high reward dependence, high harm avoidance, and low novelty seeking. Loss of control drinkers are often described as emotionally dependent, rigid, perfectionistic, anxious, inactive, quiet, patient, and introverted.

In contrast, alcohol-seeking behavior (type 2) is associated with the reverse of these traits, as seen in antisocial personalities: high novelty seeking, low harm avoidance, and low reward dependence. Type 2 alcoholics are thus described as impulsive, aggressive, impatient, confident, talkative, active, and sometimes antisocial.

Testing Predictions of the Personality Theory in a Prospective Study

Four predictions can be directly tested by a prospective longitudinal study. First, personality variation in childhood has a three-dimensional structure that corresponds to the three-dimensional structure of personality in adults. This structure is hypothesized to be moderately heritable and stable, though personality does change within limits in response to experience. Secondly, in a heterogeneous sample from the general population, the risk of alcohol abuse is predicted to increase with deviation from the mean of each of three dimensions in both high and low direction. This bidirectional effect occurs because a heterogeneous sample includes both type 1 and type 2 alcoholics, and only individuals who are average on all three dimensions are resistant to both patterns of response to alcohol. Thirdly, the risk of alcohol abuse is expected to increase exponentially rather than linearly with deviation from the mean. The non-linearity of the risk function is expected because susceptibility of alcohol abuse is hypothesized to involve failure of neurophysiological adaptive mechanisms to maintain homeostasis in response to alcohol. The failure of homeostatic control in such developmental negative feedback systems usually increases more rapidly than the linear function of underlying liability.

By making ratings of personality in childhood (11 years) rather than in adolescence, we tried to insure that the personality traits are antecedents of alcohol abuse (Cloninger et al., 1988). The four specified predictions of the theory were tested in a prospective longitudinal study of children who had detailed behavioral assessments at age 11 and who were evaluated for later misuse of alcohol at age 27.

Subjects

This study was part of a prospective longitudinal study of children who were registered for adoption in Stockholm in a two-year period during the 1950s. A total of 624 children were so registered by their mothers with the child welfare authorities of the City of Stockholm. At age 11, 431 children had been followed up for a detailed behavioral assessment including a semi-structured interview with their class teachers (Bohman, 1971).

A predefined rating key described the behaviors characteristic of each rating level on each variable; this rating key was adopted from the Berkeley Growth Study (MacFarlane et al., 1954). A short summary of the interview with descriptive examples of the child's behavior was prepared by the interviewer. These ratings and narrative summaries were used to rate childhood personality dimensions according to the theory outlined previously on a seven-point scale (Cloninger et al., 1988).

Evaluations of alcohol abuse through age 27 were prepared independently, by means of registrations with the Temperance Boards, arrests for drunkenness or driving while intoxicated, treatment for alcoholism or its complications, or a psychiatric diagnosis of alcoholism.

Classification of Personality Dimensions

The teacher ratings were really ordinal level data, with difference between adjacent scores having different behavior significance in different parts of the range of each variable. These ratings and the narrative summaries of the interviewers were used to make ratings of the three theoretically defined dimensions of novelty seeking, harm avoidance, and reward dependence. More detailed descriptions of the dimensions and their interactions are presented elsewhere for adults; they were found to be equally applicable to children (Cloninger et al., 1988).

Personality Scale Effects and Risk of Alcohol Abuse

Among the 233 boys, 30 had been registered for alcohol abuse at age 27. Only 2 of the 198 girls had been registered. As can be seen in Table 2, the risk of alcohol abuse is related to the childhood personality ratings, with personality divided simply into three groups; high, average, and low.

Table 2. Childhood personality and alcohol abuse in young adults.

Childhood personality rating	Boys N	Later Alcohol Abuse (%)	Relative Risk*
Harm avoidance			
High	70	10	0.7
Average	99	9	0.5
Low	64	22	2.7**
Novelty seeking			
High	89	19	2.4**
Average	101	11	0.7
Low	43	5	0.3
Reward dependence			
High	97	14	1.3
Average	89	8	0.4***
Low	47	19	1.9

*Relative risk is ratio of risk of the specified group to the risk in the total population.
**Boys with low harm avoidance or high novelty seeking have greater risk of later alcohol abuse than other boys ($p<0.05$).
***Boys with average reward dependence have a lower risk of later alcohol abuse than other boys ($p=0.07$).

As expected for an early-onset group, the risk of alcohol abuse was increased in individuals with the traits associated with antisocial personality: high novelty seeking, low harm avoidance, and low reward dependence.

However, further analysis showed that the risk of alcoholism was a non-linear function of the personality deviations. Although there was a predominant influence of low harm avoidance and high novelty seeking, the risk of alcoholism increased exponentially with deviations from average values to either high or low poles of each of the three dimensions, which is illustrated in Table 3.

Table 3. Quantitative personality deviations and non-linearity of risk for later alcohol abuse.

Childhood personality rating	Boys N	Later Alcohol Abuse (%)	Risk Ratio*
Harm avoidance			
+2 or +3	21	14	1.6
+1	49	8	0.9
0	99	9	1.0
-1	39	18	2.0
-2 or -3	25	28	3.1
Novelty seeking			
+2 or +3	65	25	2.3
+1	24	4	0.4
0	101	11	1.0
-1	27	0	0.0
-2 or -3	16	13	1.2
Reward dependence			
+2 or +3	30	20	2.5
+1	67	12	1.5
0	89	8	1.0
-1	29	17	2.2
-2 or -3	18	22	2.8

*Risk ratio is ratio of risk of the specified group to the risk in the total population.

These two childhood variables alone distinguished boys who had nearly twenty-fold differences in their risk of future alcohol abuse: the risk of abuse varied from 4% to 75% depending on childhood personality (Cloninger et al., 1988).

Summary

All of the predictions made were confirmed by this prospective risk study, providing strong support for the neurobiological learning theory of susceptibility to alcoholism we have proposed here. Personality in childhood has a three-dimensional structure similar to that observed elsewhere in adults. Absolute

228 Michael Bohman, C. Robert Cloninger, Sören Sigvardsson

deviations from the mean values of each of the three dimensions of childhood personality are associated with an exponential increase in the risk of later alcohol abuse.

We found three largely independent dimensions of personality at 11 years which were predictive of alcohol abuse in young adults. We also found that motor activity, impulsiveness, and poor concentration were strongly correlated. High novelty seeking and low harm avoidance were most strongly associated with alcohol abuse in young adults. Because of their youth, these alcoholics are also expected to be predominantly type 2 alcoholics. But absolute deviations in all three personality traits were also significantly associated with risk of alcohol abuse, as predicted for a heterogeneous sample. For instance, high harm avoidance, i.e., personalities characterized by high psychic anxiety, were associated with high risk of abuse.

The personality traits such as we have described here have consistently been found to have heritabilities between 40% and 60%, so that genetic and environmental factors have roughly equal importance in the development of adaptive personality traits overall. Personality certainly accounts for a substantial part of the heritable risk for alcoholism, but other biogenetic risk factors are probably also important.

References

Berger, M. (1982). Personality development and temperament. *Ciba Foundation Symposium, 89,* 176–190.

Bohman, M. (1970). *Adopted children and their families.* Stockholm: Proprius.

Bohman, M. (1971). A comparative study of adopted children, foster children and children in their biological environment born after undesired pregnancies. *Acta Paediatrica Scandinavica, Suppl. 221,* 5–38.

Bohman, M., Sigvardsson, S., & Cloninger, C. R. (1981). Maternal inheritance of alcohol abuse. *Archives of General Psychiatry, 38,* 965–969.

Cloninger, C. R. (1987). A systematic method for clinical description and classification of personality variants. *Archives of General Psychiatry, 44,* 573–588.

Cloninger, C. R., Bohman, M., & Sigvardsson, S. (1981). Inheritance of alcohol abuse: Cross-fostering analysis of adopted men. *Archives of General Psychiatry, 38,* 861–868.

Cloninger, C. R., Sigvardsson, S., & Bohman, M. (1988). Childhood personality predicts alcohol abuse in young adults. *Alcoholism: Clinical & Experimental Research*. In press.

Eysenck, S. B., & Long, F. Y. (1986). A cross-cultural comparison of personality in adults and children: Singapore and England. *Journal of Personality and Social Psychology, 50,* 124–130.

Goldsmith, H. H. (1983). Genetic influences on personality from infancy to adulthood. *Child Development, 54,* 331–355.

Loehlin, J. C. (1982). Are personality traits differentially heritable? *Behaviour Genetics, 12,* 417–428.

MacFarlane, J. W., Allen, L., & Honzik, M. P. (1954). *A development study of the behavior problems of normal children between twenty-one months and fourteen years.* Berkeley, CA: University of California Press.

Olweus, D. (1980). The consistency issue in personality psychology revisited—With special reference to aggression. *British Journal of Social and Clinical Psychology, 19,* 377–390.

Tellegen, A. (1985). Structures of mood and personality and their relevance to assessing anxiety, with an emphasis on self-report. In A. Tuma, & J. Maser (Eds.), *Anxiety and the anxiety disorders* (pp. 681–706). Hillsdale, NJ: Erlbaum.

Prediction and Prevention

Yannis Tsiantis

The need for prevention in matters of the mental health and psychosocial development of the child and the relationship between prediction and prevention constitute a promising field for the development of research into issues of child and adolescent psychiatry. Professor Bohman's work (Bohman, this volume) is impressive, and there are many interesting points in it, some of which I will refer to. It offers a theoretical model of personality structure in relation to genetic factors which could account for susceptibility to alcohol abuse. It is claimed, in other words, that personality traits account for a substantial part of the heritable risk of alcoholism in the population studied. This theory, referring to the extent to which inheritance of personality accounts for the inheritance of susceptibility to alcohol abuse, has a neurobiological basis, and it is related to structures of the brain responsible for neuroadaptive mechanisms. The time span of this longitudinal study is an impressive one, as it covers a period of 20 years. It also provides an opportunity for discussion of aspects of the prediction–prevention relationship.

One general issue is whether it is possible to use prospective risk studies of this type to determine target variables that could be used as a basis for investigating the possibility of carrying out preventive intervention. Research into questions of prevention in the mental health of children and adolescents is an enormous field and includes a wide range of investigative methods. At one extreme is basic research, which provides new knowledge concerning the causation of the various disorders of the mental health and psychosocial development of the child. We are all familiar with the view that multifactorial causation models are the rule in most of the psychosocial disorders of childhood. The results of such research work, however, can have only remote applications for decisions about actual prevention program implementation. At the other extreme is evaluative research, which assesses whether a program is effective in relation to its goals. Research of this type helps us to decide whether or not the program ought to be continued, but it cannot help us to gather a better understanding of the nature of the disorder or the processes by which it was prevented from occurring, without further research to test the generality of program effects or to pinpoint the most crucial components of the program.

When we talk of preventive action in the field of mental health, we use definitions implemented in the practice of public health, that is, primary, secondary, and tertiary prevention. Primary prevention refers to measures intended to avert the appearance of disease or impairment and thus to reduce the incidence. Secondary prevention includes all measures to promote the early diagnosis of disease and the use of effective medical treatment or other measures to shorten the duration of illness, to reduce the danger of relapse and to limit sequelae, thus reducing the prevalence. Tertiary prevention deals with chronic disease that has passed beyond the point at which available methods permit the return of the individual to full health. It thus includes all methods that limit disability and promote maximal physiological and psychological functions in patients with irreversible disease (Eisenberg, 1962).

It could be said that the most interesting and challenging aspect of preventive actions is that of primary prevention: primary preventive action aimed at eliminating the causes of dysfunction and action intended to promote health through the development of positive competences.

On the other hand, secondary preventive action will depend to a large extent on how far it is possible to deliver effective forms of treatment to all those in need. This presupposes the existence of treatment structures, and it should also be noted that special emphasis should be given to identifying and reaching untreated cases in the community.

Since the pioneering work of G. Kaplan, there has been great enthusiasm for the potential of primary prevention. But today we must accept that primary prevention calls for a very pragmatic and cautious approach, together with a constant readiness to submit promising hypotheses to the test of empirical research. It should be borne in mind that primary prevention encompasses two aspects: specific prevention and health promotion.

Special Issues

I should now like to draw attention to a number of further points which, I think, are of practical importance and bear implications for prediction research through prospective risk studies and for prevention experiments, particularly in primary prevention. In other words, I shall not confine myself to the subject of specific predictions derived from a neurobiological learning theory about the role of heritable personality traits in susceptibility to alcohol abuse.

1. It has been said that most psychosocial disorders of childhood appear to have multifactorial causation, which makes it extremely difficult to find causal relationships between causative factors and the eventual disorder. It is therefore important to adopt *multifactorial causation models in conceptualizing prevention activities.*

It has been said, of course, that a knowledge of the risk factors does not mean that people will act in such a way as to avert the consequences. There are advantages in conceptualizing prevention activities in terms of multiple risk factor orientation. This view introduces the concept that our intervention experiments to reduce the incidence of dysfunctional behavior could take place on a number of levels (multilevel intervention).

Thus, for example, preventive action may be aimed at reducing the impact of environmental stress at community or familial levels, or the intervention programs may be intended to reinforce the individual's ability to cope with stress. This issue is one of empirical benefit: which form of intervention has the best results at the lowest cost.

2. We all know that in prevention we are talking about high-risk groups, and that much preventive action is aimed at these groups. We are also familiar with the idea that children are members of a high-risk group not only because of certain features they may have, but because in daily life they may face circumstances that make demands on their adaptability that they are unable to meet effectively. It follows that preventive action may be directed either at the environment (*risk situations*) or at the children involved (*risk groups*).

In the first of these two instances, the purpose is to change the risk situation or event in the environment, and in the second to strengthen the coping styles of the children so that they can deal effectively with new problems as these arise after exposure to stress.

In evaluating the probability of the risk, using the multiple risk factor principle, it is essential to assess "How high is the risk?" This is not only done by identifying the various risk factors, but is also possible by assessing the individual significance of each one. The planning, implementation, and evaluation of specific intervention experiments aimed at modifying each of the risk factors lie on a second level. It is also necessary to investigate and analyze the effectiveness of the various combinations of individual intervention actions.

3. Another question I would like to touch on concerns the problems that arise when the intervention is designed to *prevent low baserate disorders* in the general population. If we are talking about alcoholism, for instance, problem drinking is estimated to occur in some countries in 10% of the general population and serious alcoholism in 3%. The problems emerging in these cases when implementing prevention programs could be as follows:

— the difficulty of finding a large enough number of cases to form a risk group;

— regardless of the methodology used and even with well-selected and well-planned methods of preventive intervention aimed at low baserate disorders, it is difficult to produce statistically significant results because we need a large number of subjects to which to apply the methods.

4. Longitudinal risk research provides an opportunity for examining the differing course of development of the high-risk children and the control group and especially of those children who, while at high risk, in the end do not develop the disorder (Garmezy, 1974). I am referring, in other words, to *developmental psychopathology*. Professor Bohman's research work identified three personality factors—high novelty seeking, low harm avoidance, and reward dependence—as predictive of later alcohol abuse; high novelty seeking and low harm avoidance were most strongly predictive of early-onset alcohol abuse. These personality traits manifest themselves with typical behavior patterns. Could these traits be the target variables?

Obviously, of course, other factors such as the coping styles and lifestyles of the individuals, familial and social factors, life events, and the complex interrelationship between them could all be seen as predisposing factors in addition to those mentioned above, and they could contribute to the eventual abuse of alcohol.

One crucial question is why individuals with the same personality traits do not all develop the same tendency toward alcohol abuse. We could hypothesize that these other individuals have some protective factor or mechanism, but it would be better to approach the whole issue through an investigative process taking the developmental perspective as a point of reference.

It has been proposed that the objective of this effort should be to expand research work on psychopathology with the focus not so much on the identification of characteristics, behavior, or symptoms, or of personality traits in childhood, but rather on the individual's *adaptation patterns* and particularly on a certain *adaptational failure* that could be defined in terms of crucial issues related to specific developmental tasks at a given age period. Sroufe and Rutter claim that "regardless of whether particular patterns of early adaptation or maladaptation are to a greater or lesser extent influenced by inherent dispositions or by early experience, they are nonetheless the patterns of adaptation or maladaptation" (Sroufe & Rutter, 1984, p. 23).

In line with the above, the study of adaptation development in selected individuals who do not manifest disorders—in this case the individuals who do not indulge in alcohol abuse—would be of great interest because it would help to identify possible protective factors or suitable adaptational patterns.

It has been said that the field of research which is concerned with the investigation of protective factors is a most promising one, since some individuals—although belonging to a high-risk group—do not manifest disordered behavior. It is essential for this that we acquire a more profound knowledge of the developmental processes, especially of which are the crucial issues that are related to developmental tasks at any specific age, since only then will it be possible to study the separate and individual ways of adaptation and possible maladaptation (Sroufe & Rutter, 1984).

It is important that we assume the adaptation process for each child to consist of both cognitive and affective components. We should also bear in mind the demands of the environment on the child and, more generally, the environmental changes that go on around the child, not forgetting that assimilation of the new environment and experiences will be related to the adaptational history of the child. I am making a plea for the feeling of the children and for the way in which the children interpret and assimilate new experiences on the basis of their current life situation and their past experiences and life events.

This point of view contains the issues of continuity and change of behavior raised by Kagan (1984), according to whom development does not consist of a series of linear accretions, but of a reorganization of older and newer elements (Kagan, 1984). In Professor Bohman's work, the two childhood personality factors alone, high novelty seeking and low harm avoidance, distinguish boys who had nearly 20-fold differences in their risk of alcohol abuse.

This vulnerability may perhaps be explained on the basis of the hypothesis that boys are biologically more at risk—in other words, that boys have some predisposing factors—and/or that this is combined with the presence of specific provoking or precipitating factors. This, of course, raises a general question as to our strategy for the preventive experiments: Will such intervention be directed toward preventing this vulnerability by protecting the individual against the predisposing factors (primary prevention)? Or will it also be applied to prevention of frank morbidity in vulnerable children, protecting them against the provoking factors (secondary prevention)?

Clearly, there can be no fixed strategy boundaries as regards primary or secondary prevention experiments: One tends to merge into the other as the the life-cycle evolves.

5. We should remember, on the other hand, that our research approach to preventive intervention should take account of *ecology*, which involves investigation of our relationship and transactions with our environment and the manner in which this relationship can affect human adaptation.

Ecology is concerned with the social group and its characteristics in the sense that they have a life and a force of their own. One of the aims of ecology is to discover ways of organizing the environment so as to allow individuals to develop in the best possible manner (Moos, 1976; Bronfenbrenner, 1979).

One simple example of the intervention of this type is *school,* and research has produced a considerable body of evidence that the school has a significant effect on the behavior and academic performance of children (Moos & Moos, 1978; Rutter et al., 1979). Undoubtedly, however, intervention in the social environment of the child, even at the level of the school classroom, presents quite a number of difficulties. One of the issues for which provision must be made is that after the implementation of a preventive intervention in a social group, different children may react in different ways, and this different manner of reaction may be maladaptive for some of them.

Evidence to date, however, has provided us with the contours of a very complicated set of factors that influence the nature of the social context, including the qualities of children, the characteristics and goals of the setting and larger environmental and organizational context within which that smaller setting is contained.

6. The importance of *social support* and its health-protective efforts are well known, and therefore in preventive activities work can be done through the natural support systems with the use of individual consultation, institutional consultation, or mental health education (Heller & Swindle, 1983). However, the problem that remains to be resolved in these situations in order to evaluate research activities is that of what exactly happens. We know, for instance, that social organizational factors influence the behavior of children at school. Findings suggest that schools act as an influence for good (or bad), even when children come from impoverished backgrounds. That, however, is not the same as saying that the effect of the social group modified children's responses to stressors. This point needs to be studied (Rutter, 1981). Nor do we know whether health protection is a factor of access to an optimal number of social ties, or whether certain types of social ties are implicated in maintaining people's physical and psychological well-being. It is not known which resources can be transmitted from one person to another and which are capable of moderating the stress that might otherwise overwhelm people. Some further issues in this connection are as follows:

— *Early case identification,* with or without effective preventive efforts, may have systemic implications throughout the entire ecological network. One known effect is the labeling process. This raises ethical problems as well as political issues—and general concerns about human rights and the invasion of privacy—such as the degree of responsibility that society passes to individuals for their problems or how far mental health professionals have the right to intrude into families if there is no request or formal consent for intervention.

— *Reaching the risk group* or finding the outreach cases and outreach programs may be called for to identify untreated cases of psychological disorder or risk groups that are unknown to the treatment services. Furthermore, even if one is able to identify these cases and overcome the ethical issues, some of the cases may refuse to accept help.

It has been suggested that one of the basic issues in designing prevention activities is not only the question of precise methodology, but also the definition and enlistment of high-risk groups. How one defines and gains access to the high-risk population to be served will in effect determine whether efforts are targeted or scattered, regardless of whether those reached are actually at risk or just willing participants. It is known that one way out of this situation is to develop a systematic connection between the risk group and an existing service team.

7. Another question relates to the people *who use health services* and, particularly, to our awareness that quite often the people who use the mental health services are those who have the least need of them. In practice, that is, the high-risk group never comes in contact with the services because it may find the various support systems provided by the community in which it lives adequate (McKinlay, 1972, 1973). One important factor in whether or not those in need use the mental health services is the way in which the natural social environment interacts with the existing service environment to determine, on a joint basis, the way in which people in need may make use of the services.

Research has produced considerable evidence that the use of mental health services by people in need depends on the characteristics of the social network—size, density, composition, etc.—and the functions of the social networks in the following areas: access to and diffusion of new information (the network as communication system), formation and expression of social norm conformity pressure (the network as referral system), buffer against stress (the network as support system), and problem-oriented support and advice (the network as support system) (Gottlieb & Hall, 1980).

Consequently, it could be said that social network research has invaluable potential as a means for the analysis and improvement of the relationship between the community primary mental health or primary health care group and a formal service program. This is an important point, because—apart from anything else—it will help to develop a better relationship between specialist mental health agencies and the primary health care services.

Conclusions

To conclude, longitudinal risk research is a very powerful tool for the study of causal processes and determining the precursors that may predict later pathology or disordered behavior in adult life.

Determination of the risk factors will allow us to identify the population at risk and/or risk situations that may be expected to lead to vulnerability. This determination is essential in setting the goals of our preventive intervention. I have also discussed the position according to which it is important to expand research work in search of protective factors, in relation, too, with the adaptation patterns of the individual, principally toward specific adaptational failure, which could be defined in terms of the crucial issues related to the developmental tasks of a given age period.

I have suggested that it is important to adopt a multifactorial causation model in conceptualizing prevention activities, and I have proposed that multilevel intervention is quite often necessary.

I have looked into some issues relating to the difficulties in identifying the high-risk groups and generally in establishing outreach programs, with emphasis on the ethical issues involved and wider concerns of human rights and the invasion of privacy.

References

Bronfenbrenner, U. (1979). *The ecology of human development: Experiments by nature and design.* Cambridge, MA: Harvard University Press.

Eisenberg, L. (1962). Preventive psychiatry. *Annual Review of Medicine, 13,* 343–360.

Garmezy, N. (1974). The study of competence in children at risk for severe psychopathology. In E. J. Anthony & C. Koupernik (Eds.), *The child in his family, Vol. 3.* New York: Wiley.

Gottlieb, B., & Hall, A. (1980). Social networks and the utilization of preventive mental health services. In R. Price, R. Ketterer, B. Bader, & J. Monahan (Eds.), *Prevention in mental health* (Sage Annual Reviews of Community Mental Health, Vol. 1) (pp. 167–194). Beverly Hills/London: Sage.

Heller, K., & Swindle, R. (1983). Social networks, perceived social support and coping with stress. In R. Felner, J. Leonard, J. Moritsugu, & S. Farber (Eds.), *Preventive psychology*. New York: Pergamon.

Kagan, J. (1984). *The nature of the child*. New York: Basic Books.

McKinlay, J. (1972). Some approaches and problems in the study of the use of services. An overview. *Journal of Health and Social Behavior, 13,* 115–151.

McKinlay, J. (1973). Social networks, lay consultation and helping behavior. *Social Forces, 51,* 275–292.

Moos, R. H. (1976). *The human context: Environmental determination of behavior*. New York: Wiley.

Moos, R. H., & Moos, B. (1978). Classroom social climate and students' absences and grades. *Journal of Educational Psychology, 20,* 263–269.

Rutter, M., Maughan, B., Mortimore, P., Ouston, J., & Smith, A. (1979). *Fifteen thousand hours: Secondary schools and their effects on children*. London: Open Books.

Rutter, M. (1981). Stress, coping and development: Some issues and some questions. *Journal of Child Psychology and Psychiatry, 22,* 323–356.

Sroufe, A., & Rutter, M. (1984). The domain of developmental psychopathology. *Child Development, 55,* 17–29.

Prevention Research on Early Risk Behaviors in Cross-Cultural Studies

Sheppard G. Kellam, James C. Anthony,
C. Hendricks Brown, Lawrence Dolan,
Lisa Werthamer-Larsson, Renate Wilson

Behavioral responses in childhood are strong predictors of later developmental and psychopathological outcomes. In a major review of the literature linking childhood behavior to adult disorder, Kohlberg and colleagues (1984) concluded that global indicators of childhood maladaptation (e.g., school failure, poor peer relations, antisocial behavior) predict adult disorder. Early aggressiveness and antisocial behavior are strong indicators of later criminality and drug use, especially in boys (Conger & Miller, 1966; Farrington, 1978; Mitchell & Rosa, 1981; Robins, 1966, 1978). Kellam et al. (1980) and Ensminger et al. (1983) found this predictive relationship to be enhanced when aggressive boys were also rated high on the shy component of behavior. We defined aggressive behavior as fighting and breaking rules, and shy behavior as not raising one's hand, and sitting and playing alone. These behavioral responses have been found to be important early predictors in our developmental epidemiological research in Woodlawn (Kellam et al., 1983, 1982).

Early behavioral responses, which are the focus of particular attention in the work of the Johns Hopkins Prevention Research Center (PRC), must be studied biologically, socially, and psychologically in order to understand their origins and their functions on the developmental paths leading to psychopathology and antisocial outcomes. Preventive trials carried out in Baltimore, Maryland, in the form of field experiments are directed at changing particular behaviors in the interest of determining whether the risk of specific later problem outcomes is reduced. Periodic outcome evaluations of the two Baltimore PRC trials have both a theoretical and a utilitarian aim: The former will provide data on the changeability of early risk behaviors and their etiologic significance for outcomes, while the latter is concerned with improving risk.

In the Woodlawn studies, conducted in Chicago from 1963 to the present, we conceptualized mental health as having two distinctly measurable components (Kellam et al., 1975). The first is an internal feeling of well-being related to thought processes, affective status, self-esteem, and other aspects of individual psychological status. We term this component *psychological well-being* (PWB) and include signs, symptoms, and disorders here. The second consists of the adequacy of the individual's performance of social task demands in the major social fields appropriate to his/her stage in the life cycle. We have named this component *social adaptational status* (SAS). Natural raters in specific social fields, such as school teachers, define the social tasks and rate performance. Thus, anxiety, depression, and bizarre thoughts are examples of lacking PWB, while learning problems, shy behavior (not raising your hand, sitting alone), aggressive behavior (fighting and breaking rules, truancy), and trouble paying attention are examples of SAS in the school and classroom.

Woodlawn findings showed that as early as the start of elementary school in first grade there are clearly identifiable social adaptational and psychological antecedents leading to specific outcomes of psychopathology, delinquency, and other problem outcomes. Review of recent literature in industrial countries supports the Woodlawn results, and will be noted. Specifically, the Woodlawn findings were:

1. First-grade problems in learning, as rated by teachers on school IQ and readiness-for-school test performance, are a strong and specific predictor of teenage depressive and other symptoms among males and to a lesser extent among females (see also Rutter et al., 1970; Shaffer et al., 1979; Watt, 1974). Learning problems did not predict delinquency when aggression was controlled for.

2. A strong first-grade antecedent of teenage symptom levels in females is early psychiatric symptoms, while early symptoms did not predict teenage symptoms among males.

3. Shyness among first-grade males (but not females) clearly inhibits delinquency (and drug, alcohol, and cigarette use) at age 16 or 17. For males early shyness also predicts higher levels of teenage anxiety.

4. First-grade aggressiveness without shyness in males (not females) is a strong predictor of increased teenage delinquency (and drug, alcohol, and cigarette use). Similar findings have been supported in many studies (Conger & Miller, 1966; Kaplan, 1980; Lefkowitz et al., 1977; Mitchell & Rosa, 1981; Robins, 1973, 1978; Spivak et al., 1986). Aggressive-

ness without shyness was not related to later psychopathology in the Woodlawn data.

5. A combination of shyness and aggressiveness in first-grade males (not females) was associated with higher levels of delinquency and substance use than aggressiveness alone. This combination is very much like the DSM-III *undersocialized conduct disorder* (Kellam et al., 1982).

6. The social adaptational and psychological predictions do not generally interact in the effects on later delinquency, psychiatric symptoms, or other outcomes.

7. There are strong differences between males and females in the developmental paths leading to adolescent outcomes. Early school social adaptational behavioral responses have strong predictive power for both later social adaptation and psychological well-being among males (points 1, 3, 4, and 5), while early psychological well-being shows clear continuity with later psychological well-being for females (point 2).

These results support the usefulness of making a distinction between social adaptational status and psychological well-being. Also, separate study of these two measures and their interrelationships over time revealed developmental differences between the sexes. No less important was the emergence of the classroom as a crucially important social field where the teacher, as a natural rater, defines the tasks and grades the behavioral responses of the children as succeeding or failing at these tasks (see also Pedersen et al., 1978).

There is increasing evidence that some of the behavioral responses are related to biological characteristics that may place limits on the child's social adaptational responses. Recent prospective work by Kagan (1984) and Suomi (1987) on shy behavior suggest that a heightened sympathetic response set distinguishes shy, non-exploring offspring fairly early after birth.

Current Preventive Trials

The two preventive trials have recently been implemented by The Johns Hopkins Prevention Research Center in the Baltimore City Public Schools (Dolan et al., 1988; Werthamer-Larsson et al., 1988; Brown et al., 1988; Kellam et al., 1988). The first is directed at improving learning through an improved curriculum called *Mastery Learning*. The goal is to determine whether there is a direct effect of improving mastery of reading and other core skills on the reduction in risk of later psychiatric symptoms, particularly for depressive symptoms and possibly for depressive disorder. This trial also addressed a central developmental question, i.e., whether shy and/or aggressive behavior stems from the experience of failure or is a predisposition of the child in responding to classroom environment, regardless of academic success or failure.

Our second preventive trial is directed at reducing the levels of shy and aggressive behavior directly through a behavior management method called the *Good Behavior Game*. Evaluation of this trial will determine whether there is a reduction in the risk of later delinquency and heavy substance use, and whether there is a crossover effect on learning.

The evaluation of these two trials will aid us not only in the development of improved preventive interventions, but also in understanding the etiologic or at least developmental functions of shy behavior, aggressive behavior, and learning problems and their relationships to psychiatric symptoms and disorders.

The developmental perspective we add to the epidemiologic foundations of the two trials is important. Periodic longitudinal measures are required for understanding the development and flexibility of behavioral and psychological responses and their interrelationships as well as providing information about when to add additional intervention programs. We can determine the slopes of these effects over time by periodic assessment of the developmental effect of the two intervention trials, both in comparison to each other and to control classrooms and schools. The current plan is for a 5-year follow-up, with the likelihood of continuing assessment into adolescence and adulthood. Two cohorts of 1200 entering first-graders will have received the intervention for two years by the time of this periodic follow-up. Both cohorts will be assessed annually through sixth grade, while mothers and fathers (or surrogates) will be interviewed in fourth and sixth grades. Each year child assessments will include teacher ratings, classmate ratings, self-report, and school achievement, attendance, and grades. Parents will be interviewed concerning family structure; learning environment and behavior management; parental mental health and substance use; parent ratings of child mental health and behavior; a service or utilization. Each core construct will be measured by multiple methods. Detailed tracking and assessment procedures have been developed to follow students over time.

The Design

The core research design consisted of two first-grade cohorts of students in the Baltimore City Public Schools. The first cohort began school during the 1985–1986 academic year and the second during the 1986–1987 academic year. The two interventions were mounted over a period of two years for each cohort.

The design called for testing the two interventions in each of five sets of matched school triads. Five urban areas within Elementary District B in Eastern Baltimore were selected in the light of census tract and school catchment area statistics. Selection was made with active involvement of the Baltimore City Planning Department. Three matched schools were selected within each of the five urban areas with regard to census tract, school level, and first- and second-grade level data. Within these matched triads, one school received the *Mastery Learning* intervention, one school the *Good Behavior Game* intervention, and one school served as a *Standard Setting* control. Assignments to each group were made by a random process. Within each intervention school, standard setting classrooms (which do not receive any interventions) were included in order to control for school-level variables that might confound the evaluation of the interventions. Within each school first-grade children were randomly assigned across classrooms.

Teachers were assigned to intervention condition by a chance process, with the restriction that they intend to remain in the building at the same grade level for at least a 2-year period. Teachers were representative of current elementary teachers and were not selected for specific interest in an intervention or because of positive evaluation by principals.

Multi-Method and Multi-Stage Periodic Assessments

The methodology for prevention intervention research involves several important considerations. First, the populations should be epidemiologically defined, most often at the size and level of local communities, townships, or neighborhoods. Second, a developmental perspective is central to prevention research; it entails periodic measures of sufficient frequency to allow the developmental course to be assessed. Third, multi-stage sampling and assessments are important in bridging the gap between field assessments of total cohorts and the more extensive and detailed assessments that are necessary for measuring and understanding developmental outcomes but that can only be done in the micro-analytic laboratory. Fourth, multiple measurement methods increase the validity of assessments to be determined and provide important opportunities to examine risk behaviors and conditions as well as developmental outcomes from different perspectives.

The first-stage assessments in Baltimore that enter into the evaluation of the field trials were done periodically during interventions and annually thereafter on all children in two cohorts. They included attention to both *social adaptational status* (SAS), the measurement of the adequacy of the individual's role performance as viewed by significant others in a particular social field, and *psychological well-being* (PWB), how the individual feels, including affects, self-esteem, and psychopathology. The first-stage core assessments of all children included teacher ratings of classroom adaptation, direct observations of classroom behavior, peer ratings of social acceptance, and self-reports of anxiety and depression. Additional assessment was based on school records of educational attainment, attendance, and conduct (Werthamer-Larsson et al., 1988).

Second-stage assessments will continue on representative samples for psychiatric signs and symptoms and neuropsychological function. A representative smaller third-stage sample will provide for a thorough psychiatric diagnostic work-up.

A biostatistical methods grant, which grew out of the Prevention Research Center and was funded by National Institute of Mental Health for 5 years, is an integral component of this periodic follow-up and evaluation and will supply the resources for developing increasingly powerful biostatistical methods for examining stochastic modeling of impact over time.

The Developmental Perspective

The strong links between early classroom behavior and adolescent outcomes suggest lengthy developmental processes observable from early childhood onwards and continuing at least into mid-adolescence. Data on these intervening processes are sparse, largely because of the relative absence of longitudinal research on problems through middle childhood. The task of prediction is challenging because the manifestations of mal-adaptation may change over time, reducing the likelihood of observing isomorphic indicators at different ages (Sroufe & Rutter, 1984). Careful descriptive work, which details the changing profile of adaptation or maladaptation in developing children, is needed in order to elucidate relationships linking early to later maladaptation and to disorder.

Periodic assessments conducted through middle childhood will enable a careful tracking of both early risk behaviors, psychiatric signs and symptoms, and early manifestations of problem outcomes as they emerge and change over time. By periodically assessing multiple indicators of childhood maladaptation, the developmental course of maladaptation can be investigated despite changes in behavioral profiles. The interrelationships between social adaptation and psychological well-being can be assessed. In addition, this longitudinal approach will permit estimates of the incidence, prevalence, and time of occurrence of problem outcomes (including symptoms, disorders, heavy substance use, and delinquency) at various age levels.

As important as the tracking of outcomes is the investigation of possible protective factors which this study makes possible. Children who exhibit early risk factors but do not develop problem outcomes may be said to be resistant or resilient (Garmezy et al., 1984). The question of interest here is whether our interventions can protect children from manifesting the risk behaviors and as a result protect them from problem outcomes. Thus, data on the developmental paths and on the individual and environmental risk factors leading to psychological signs, symptoms, and disorders or social maladaptation will permit us to test models of risk and vulnerability in conjunction with psychopathology. For example, we may be able to test whether there is a detectable developmental sequence from early depressive symptoms to later symptom clusters, and finally, to diagnosable affective disorder.

The study of the interplay of behavioral responses, signs and symptoms, and diagnoses is at the very nature of understanding psychopathology itself. The DSM-III field trials have underlined the continuing difficulties in obtaining agreement about childhood disorders (Hodges & Siegel, 1985). These findings raise the question of what defines a case for child psychopathology, and how good a fit exists between empirically derived data and DSM-III categories. Some scholars (e.g., Achenbach, 1980) have stated that empirically derived syndromes offer an approach to organizing problem behaviors. Periodic epidemiological trials with a developmental perspective allow us to study the interplay, from a biopsychosocial perspective, of behaviors, symptoms and signs, and disorders to inform diagnostic nosology. The next stage of understanding how best to represent psychiatric nosologic entities will be informed by examining covariation among these behavioral responses and signs and symptoms, and assessing the relationships among the covariates that lead over time to outcomes of importance to psychopathology and mental health.

Risk behaviors and signs and symptoms that covary and interact with each other to produce significant psychopathological outcomes later on may well form the basis for the next nosology of psychiatric disorder in children and adolescents. By comparing our results to DSM-III diagnoses, we can determine how empirically derived clusters of behavior, symptoms, and signs compare to the current diagnostic formulations. Such research, coupled with preventive trials, informs our measures of impact and thereby reveals how changeable the paths leading to disorders may be, as well as indicating the role that behavior changes brought about by the interventions may play in developmental psychopathology.

Cross-Cultural Programs in the Early Assessment and Prevention of Alcohol, Drugs, and Mental Disorders

An important part of the work of the PRC relates to the workscope of the WHO Collaborating Center in the Department of Mental Hygiene. Currently, we are examining the feasibility of planning a mutual exchange of trainees and of methods of cross-cultural research related to assessment and prevention of mental and behavioral disorders in children who live in different cultures and who have different schooling experiences. The research methods and conceptualizations in the Prevention Research Center may be informed by, and in turn be of value to, investigators in other societies who are also designing and/or implementing research related to preventing behavioral and mental disorders in school children and the sequelae of these disorders in later life.

An example of such research is our present plan for substantive and methodological effort with a group of longitudinal and developmental researchers from Humboldt University, German Democratic Republic, relating (a) to the testing of construct validity and reliability of classroom observation and teacher rating concepts and instruments; and (b) to doing epidemiological and developmental research cross-culturally. So far, this effort has led to the tentative formulation of a set of cross-national research questions of relevance to the WHO focus on child populations:

1. Are types and rates of classroom maladaptive behaviors among first-grade boys and girls the same or different across different national settings? And are the distributions of types of behaviors observed by various geographic and demographic settings in each area the same or different? Do the behaviors of interest have similar or different latent structures and can they be summarized in terms of the same items? Are the constructs underlying the proposed assessment instruments similar and do they test the same behaviors?

2. Are the situational and educational contexts in which the behaviors of interest occur similar or different? Are criteria for referral to special education or special learning programs similar or different?

3. On the assumption that similar behaviors occur across cultural settings, how do they relate to symptoms and disorders, and eventually to outcomes in each setting? Is there a differential effect attached to environmental factors?

4. How well do specific behaviors or symptoms predict individual outcomes in each setting, i.e., what is their respective importance in terms of life course developmental paths?

We hope to explore these questions not only with our colleagues at Humboldt, but over a wide geographical range of national and cultural settings, including countries from various regions and at different levels of urbanization and industrialization. An instrument translation and translation validation protocol has been developed and the constructs underlying selected instruments are being independently validated in each setting.

Summary

The Prevention Research Center (PRC) in the Department of Mental Hygiene at the Johns Hopkins University School of Hygiene and Public Health is focused upon early risk behaviors of children found to be predictive of ADM disorders later in the life course. Over the last 15 years there has been growing evidence that the early behavioral responses of children, particularly to the social task demands of classroom and peer group, are important sources of prediction and help define the developmental paths leading to problem outcomes later in the life course. The work of the PRC is centered in the eastern half of Baltimore, the site of the ECA and of the earlier epidemiological and preventive trial research of this Department and of our School.

This ongoing population-based prevention trial is based upon a strong collaborative relationship between the Baltimore City Public Schools and The Johns Hopkins Prevention Research Center, a necessary partnership for this record of population and community-based research. We actively sought and obtained the support of the local community organizations and the parents of the children. Through an intensive process of identifying mutual interests, it was possible to develop and carry out multiple methods of assessment and random assignment of children to two interventions and to control classrooms over the first two school years of our two cohorts. A similar strategy was used and proved successful in the Woodlawn studies.

The behavioral responses of two cohorts of first-grade children are the focus of current epidemiologic measurement and preventive trials. One intervention is directed at reducing learning problems measured by multiple methods at the first stage, since these can predict psychiatric symptoms, particularly depression, and possibly disorders. Another intervention is aimed at reducing aggressive and shy behaviors, which have been found to predict heavy drug use and delinquency. Schools are matched in triads with control classrooms within intervention schools as well as external control schools entirely separate from the intervention schools. Children are randomly assigned to intervention or control classrooms. The trials involve two cohorts of 2,400 first-graders through the first and second years of school in 19 elementary schools.

For purposes of generalizability and validity in wider contexts, these early risk behaviors must be studied cross-culturally and the strategies of preventive programs tested in different environments. As part of our role as a WHO Collaborating Center for Research and Training, methods for these types of cross-cultural epidemiologic measurement and broader public health purposes are now being developed and will be tested in several settings.

Acknowledgments

The authors wish to acknowledge the contributions of the Baltimore community, its families and children, and the administration of the Baltimore City Public Schools. The work of the Prevention Research Center would not have been possible or successful without the active participation and continued support of the leadership, faculty, and staff of the school district and their support and guidance in our research and service enterprise. The Board of School Commissioners gave their strong endorsement. The faculty and staff of the Baltimore Public Schools have made crucial contributions; specifically Alice Pinderhughes, former Superintendent of the Baltimore City Schools has been vitally important to this project. We also wish to acknowledge the continuing support of Dr. Richard Hunter, new Superintendent of Baltimore City Public Schools. The assistance and support of Leonard Wheeler, Executive Director of Eastern District; Carla Ford, Supervisor, Office of Early Childhood Education; Craig Cutter, Staff Director Department of Education; Edward Friedlander, Associate Superintendent, Division of Instructional Support Services; Leonard Granick, Staff Director; and Meldon Hollis, President of the Baltimore City Public School Board have been vital to our project, and we wish to acknowledge their contribution.

These studies have been supported by the following grants: National Institute of Mental Health, Grant Number P50 MH38725, Epidemiologic Prevention Center for Early Risk Behavior; National Institute of Mental Health, Grant Number RO1 MH40859, Center for Prevention Research Program: Methodologic Advances; National Institute on Drug Abuse, Grant Number RO1DA04392, Etiology and Prevention of Drug Related Behavior; and contracts with Dr. Allan F. Mirsky, Chief, Laboratory of Psychology and Psychopathology at the National Institute of Mental Health for technical services to provide psychological, sociometric, and demographic data sets on a population-based sample of school children.

References

Achenbach, T. M. (1980). DSM-III in light of empirical research on the classification of child psychopathology. *Journal of the American Academy of Child Psychiatry, 19,* 395–412.

Brown, C. H., Royall, R. M., & Edelsohn, G. (1988). *Analyzing data from preventive trials: Practical solutions to handling attrition.* Paper read at the APHA, November 1988, Boston, Massachusetts.

Conger, J. J., & Miller, W. C. (1966). *Personality, social class and delinquency.* New York: Wiley.

Dolan, L., Kellam, S., & Brown, C. H. (1988). *Short term impact of two preventive interventions of early risk behaviors.* Paper presented at the APHA, November 1988, Boston, Massachusetts.

Ensminger, M. E., Kellam, S. G., & Rubin, B. R. (1983). School and family origins of delinquency: Comparisons by sex. In K.T. van Dusen & S. A. Mednick (Eds.), *Prospective studies of crime and delinquency* (pp. 73–97). Boston: Kluwer-Nijhoff.

Farrington, D. P. (1978). The family backgrounds of aggressive youths. In L. Hersov, M. Berger, & D. Shaffer (Eds.), *Aggression and antisocial behavior in childhood and adolescence.* Oxford: Pergamon Press.

Garmezy, N., Masten, A. S., & Tellegen, A. (1984). The study of stress and competence in children: A building block for developmental psychology. *Child Development, 55,* 97–111.

Hodges, K. K., & Siegel, L. J. (1985). Depression in children and adolescents. In E. E. Beckham & W. R. Leber (Eds.), *Handbook of depression: Treatment, assessment and research.* Homewood, IL: Dorsey.

Kagan, J., Reznick, J. S., Clarke, C., Snidman, N., & Garcia-Coll, C. (1984). Behavioral inhibition to the unfamiliar. *Child Development, 55,* 2212–2225.

Kaplan, H. B. (1980). *Deviant behavior in defense of self.* New York: Academic Press.

Kellam, S. G., Brown, C. H., Rubin, B. R., & Ensminger, M. E. (1983). Paths leading to teenage psychiatric symptoms and substance use: Developmental epidemiological studies in Woodlawn. In S. B. Guze, F. J. Earls, & J. E. Barrett (Eds.), *Childhood psychopathology and development* (pp. 17–51). New York: Raven Press.

Kellam, S. G., Brown, C. H., & Fleming, J. P. (1982). The prevention of teenage substance abuse: Longitudinal research and strategy. In T. J. Coates, A. L. Petersen, & C. Perry (Eds.), *Promoting adolescent health: A dialogue on research and practice* (pp. 171–200). New York: Academic Press.

Kellam, S. G., Ensminger, M. E., & Simon, M. B. (1980). Mental health in first grade and teenage drug, alcohol, and cigarette use. *Drug and Alcohol Dependence, 5,* 273–304.

Kellam, S. G., Branch, J. D., Agrawal, K. C., & Ensminger, M. E. (1975). *Mental health and going to school: The Woodlawn program of assessment, early intervention, and evaluation.* Chicago: University of Chicago Press.

Kellam, S. G., Werthamer-Larsson, L. Crockett, L., Edelsohn, G., Anthony, J., Brown, C. H., Dolan, L., Wheeler, L., & Spencer, P. (1988). *Preventive trials directed at early risk behaviors: Teacher and peer ratings of social maladaptation.* Paper presented at the APHA, November, 1988, Boston, Massachusetts.

Kohlberg, L., Ricks, D., & Snarey, J. (1984). Childhood development as a predictor of adaptation in adulthood. *Genetics Psychology Monographs, 110,* 91–172.

Lefkowitz, M. M., Eron, L. C., Walden, L. O., & Heusman, L. R. (1977). *Growing up to be violent.* New York: Pergamon Press.

Mitchell, S., & Rosa, P. (1981). Boyhood behavior problems as precursors of criminality: A fifteen-year follow-up study. *Journal of Child Psychology, 22,* 19–33.

Pedersen, E., Faucher, T. A., & Eaton, W. (1978). New perspective on the effects of first-grade teachers on children's subsequent adult status. *Harvard Educational Review, 48*(1), 131.

Robins, L. N. (1966). *Deviant children grown-up: A sociological and psychiatric study of sociopathic personality.* Baltimore: Williams and Wilkins.

Robins, L. N. (1973). *A follow-up of Vietnam drug users.* Special Action Office Monograph, Series A, No. 1, Special Action Office for Drug Abuse Prevention, Washington, DC.

Robins, L. N. (1978). *Sturdy childhood predictors of adult outcomes: Replications from longitudinal studies.* Paul Hoch award lecture. Presented at the American Psychopathological Association Meeting, Boston.

Rutter, M. L., Tizard, J., & Whitmore, K. (Eds.) (1970). *Education, health and behavior: Psychological and medical study of childhood development.* New York: Wiley.

Shaffer, D., Stokman, C., O'Connor, P. A., Shafer, S., Barmack, J. E., Hess, S., & Spaulten, D. (1979). *Early soft neurological signs and later psychopathological development.* Paper presented at the annual meeting of the Society for Life History Research in Psychopathology and Society for the Study of Social Biology, New York.

Spivak, G., Marcus, J., & Swift, M. (1986). Early classroom behaviors and later misconduct. *Developmental Psychology, 22,* 124–131.

Sroufe, A. L., & Rutter, M. (1984). The domain of developmental psychology. *Child Development, 55,* 17–29.

Suomi, S. J. (1987). Genetic and maternal contributions to individual differences in rhesus monkey biobehavioral development. In N. Krasnagor (Ed.), *Psychobiological aspects of behavioral development.* Orlando, FL: Academic Press.

Watt, N. F. (1974). Childhood and adolescent routes to schizophrenia. In D. F. Ricks, A. Thomas, & M. Roff (Eds.), *Life history research in psychopathology, Volume 3* (pp. 194–211). Minneapolis: University of Minnesota Press.

Werthamer-Larsson, L., Kellam, S. G., Brown, C. H., Dolan, L., & Wheeler, L. (1988). *The epidemiology of maladaptive behavior in first grade children.* Paper presented at the APHA, November, 1988, Boston, Massachusetts.

Strategies for Prevention Research

Jon Rolf

Introduction

Prevention research, more than basic epidemiological and clinical research must be an integrative, interdisciplinary field. From the literature, it is clear that prevention researchers are learning from trial and error. The longer a particular area of prevention or health promotion research has existed, the more refined the research designs have become. Even so, one finds a dominance of simplistic causal models inadequately controlled, non-randomized, quasi-experimental designs presently being used. There are a number of reasons why prevention research remains unsophisticated. It's partly because of the philosophical prejudices of early prevention advocates. Part of the problem lies in the difficulty in creating testable prevention models from the complex integrative, multifactorial theories involving relevant "development of persons in contexts" perspectives. No doubt, some of the problems in advancing prevention research lie in the ethical and pragmatic difficulties of implementing prevention research in field settings. And some portion of the problem is a result of insufficient numbers of adequately trained investigators who are motivated and able to effect multidisciplinary collaborations.

In spite of these problems, progress is being made in finding better strategies for improving prevention research. My task is to outline some of them. It would seem that the scope of this task is better suited to a monograph than to a rather short presentation. However, if I leave many of the details aside, I can sketch in some of the problems and their potential remedies.

Countering Old Prejudices and Value Orientations

Experience has taught us that it is very difficult to know how to adapt the very best theories and methods from each of the parent disciplines in designing prevention research. The depth and breadth of experience, moreover, differ between areas of preventive intervention research for psychopathology and physical health problems. For example, there has been more sustained effort in preventive intervention research for cardiac disease in adults and conduct learning problems in school-aged children. There has been a substantial amount of work and even more rhetoric concerning alcohol and other substance abuse prevention efforts with adolescents. There has been relatively little work in other areas such as child abuse, disaster-induced stress disorders, and even fewer attempts to prevent such specific psychopathologies as depressive disorders in early adolescence. The reasons for these different degrees of effort and progress are more a result of policy and philosophy than the prevalence of seriousness of the disorders in need of prevention.

I will begin by mentioning three philosophical orientations espoused by pioneers in the prevention field which still leave unresolved tensions inhibiting interdisciplinary and inter-specialty cooperations. The three are

— jealous competition with established treatment systems,

— hostility concerning the relative value of promotion vs prevention,

— dogmatism about equating "true" primary prevention with mass-targeted as compared to research models targeting high-risk groups.

In the late 1980s, it is important to recognize that the primary prevention literature has already been overburdened with too much rhetoric and too much polarization by its early advocates and detractors.

Complementing not Combatting the Treatment System

Several authors have reviewed the various ways that prevention research in the United States has been shaped by politics and policy decisions in the service delivery systems and the research support institutions (e.g., Roberts & Peterson, 1984). They point to evidence that prevention research has been handicapped by the "treatment mentality" dominating mental health value concepts. This mentality is reinforced by two factors: First, the difficulty of refuting the logic that, given limited resources, one should expend them on already disturbed persons in need of treatment; second, the mental health service delivery system is dependent on a cost-recovery system based on the treatment of disorders. In the United States, only the relatively few health maintenance organizations (HMOs) with prepaid health fees are interested in preventive services that might reduce their clients' need for treatment delivery. The majority of treatment institutions, however, are not willing to spend resources for prevention efforts that would not be recoverable through medical insurance.

Many of the early advocates for prevention recommended that prevention researchers break away from the treatment system and distance themselves as much as possible from treatment paradigms. For example, one should avoid targeting interventions for persons too close to the brink of diagnosable disorders. This resembled early treatment and could at best be "secondary prevention." The dogma of the early prevention advocates was clear: True prevention must be primary prevention, and primary prevention, by definition, must be delivered to persons who have not even begun to show the early symptoms of the onset of the targeted disorder. These early prevention advocates also insisted that true primary prevention must be "mass-targeted," that is, delivered in uniform doses to healthy persons in the general population. More suspect were selective approaches designed for intervention with specific groups at high risk who could be served in conjunction with an already established treatment institution.

Thus, emphasis on health promotion assured avoidance of contamination of primary prevention with treatment. Consequently, educative and competency-building programs were recommended by early prevention advocates for implementation in schools and at the community level. Such approaches would, of course, also net both the most highly vulnerable and the less vulnerable non-disordered persons in order to promote greater coping skills and to improve well-being. The reduction of the future incidence of treatable psychopathology was desirable but not immediately necessary.

Common Sense Solutions

Today, common sense can resolve the old value dilemmas in order to promote more attitudes toward prevention research. The basic options are shown in Table 1. Broad categories of intervention subjects can be given experimental preventive in-

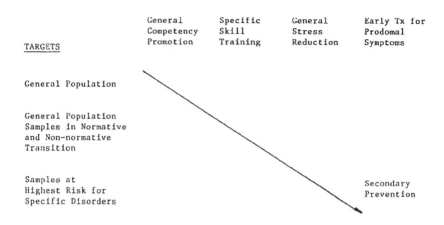

Table 1. Broad categories of preventive intervention and targets.

terventions complementary, but not replicating or competing with services traditionally available in systems treating mental disorders.

For example, there is no need to re-argue the ideal formula for determining how much general promotion of competencies must be included in "true" primary prevention research. Any prevention research project has the potential to demonstrate effects of prevention: the reduction of negative outcomes and promotion of increased quantity of health-enhancing behaviors and enhanced qualities of life. It seems more reasonable to evaluate future prevention research efforts on

a) the extent to which the intervention model successfully combined intervention elements for health promotion and disorder prevention;

b) how many of the outcome variables target the quantitative and qualitative aspects of negative and positive outcomes.

Coping with Public Health Professionals' Neglect of Health Promotion

The roots of preventive intervention research go back to the fields of public health and clinical approaches to the treatment of individuals with illnesses. The fields differ in that the public health is population-based and the clinical tradition is individual-based. Today, it is certainly true that the public health model is dominated by epidemiology and actuarial methods designed to count cases and to identify potentially predictive risk and protective factors. Surprisingly, very few experimental health promotion intervention studies are conducted by public health researchers. This may well be a result of a host of reasons. But chief among this is the paucity of behavioral scientists who are able to tackle the behavioral habits and psychological processes that, at the same time, are (1) the most prevalent population-based health risks in developed countries and (2) processes not amenable to medical-model "magic bullet pharmacological or vaccine risk-reduction methods."

Epidemiology Is an Easily Mastered and Currently Necessary Tool for Large-Scale Prevention Research

Many important new public health prevention programs will be based on behavioral rather than biological sciences. Mental health researchers will doubtlessly play key roles in their development. Even so, prevention and health-promotion researchers who endeavor to extend behavioral change methodology to society's current public health problems cannot afford to ignore the traditional expectations by public health professionals that epidemiological and actuarial risk statistics must always form the basis for targeting high-risk groups, planning large-scale interventions, and in reporting results in terms of morbidity and mortality.

This point is well illustrated by the NIH response to the AIDS epidemic in the United States. For several years, no funds were designated for behaviorally based prevention efforts directed at the general population because epidemiological data indicated that it was currently then actuarially at low risk. Some very limited funds for preventive efforts were directed toward the highest risk groups (homosexuals and intravenous drug users), but the vast majority of research budgets were for further epidemiology, i.e., risk assessment of potential hosts, and for virology, i.e., understanding the biological agent. The attitude among most public health policymakers was that it is less important to study methods to block behavioral transmission of HIV. Further, it would be ridiculous to devote any funds toward the prevention of HIV infection among normal adolescents because they were not at high actuarial risk.

The fallacy of this actuarial-distorted logic is now clear to almost everyone in public health research. However, it does indicate that funding will for the present be available for prevention research targeting only extremely high-risk groups regardless of whether or not there are sufficiently potent interventions to alter their health-risking behavior. Strategies to cope with mismatches between risk potency and that of the experimental intervention are discussed more fully in a subsequent section.

Developmental Perspectives

Prevention researchers are learning that one can't live with them or without them.

Even though the etiology of most psychopathologies is not well understood at present, there would probably be consensus among clinical researchers that the causal chains are complex and probably span a number of years during which developmental processes are important determinants of behavior. Etiological theories often contain provision for *critical periods* during which the individual is most sensitive toward pathogenic influences or for entering developmental pathways that may lead to disordered adult outcomes. Since prevention researchers cannot hope to conduct their studies during the often long periods when vulnerable individuals may be capable of developing the targeted psychopathology, they will often attempt to select a particularly early or transitional developmental period that appears to be the most risky one for failing to adapt successfully to its inherent developmental challenges.

Epidemiologic data can be helpful in bracketing critical periods appropriate to short-term preventive intervention research. For example, increases in stress-related disorders, suicidal ideation, and depression symptoms can be shown by large-scale surveys to increase during the transition from structured elementary school to the less uniformed tracking of junior high school and high school. Unfortunately, however, there is really very little data on the normative patterns of adjustment, adaptive responses to life stressors during life development, and longitudinal patterns of risk expression that could provide what Cowen (1980) says is needed for a solid generative data base for persons embarking on confirmatory preventive intervention research for youthful subjects (Garmezy & Rutter, 1983).

Earlier Is Not Always Better

Among the major reasons why prevention and promotion research has often been directed at very young children is the supposition that early preventive interventions are more likely to be more effective than interventions given at a later time. (Zigler and Berman [1983], for example, reviewed the importance of hypothesized critical periods during infancy for developmental deficit in the advocacy of strategies that lead to legislating the Head Start day-care programs in the United States.) We also find that researchers interested in the prevention of sociopathy often chose to implement preventive interventions targeting conduct disorders in school-aged children who are entering a "critical period" of developmental challenge involved in transitioning from parental to peer group authority structures. Similarly, substance-abuse prevention researchers often target early adolescents to test their preventive interventions during this developmental period with its high normative rates of risky behaviors, including experimentation with drugs, that are initiated and evaluated by peer groups. In these latter cases, earlier is not automatically better. This is because intervention effects become too difficult to prove as a function of longer assessment time spans and the more dissimilar the proximal behavior is to the distal diagnosable criterion condition.

Prevention Research Design Options

Prevention researchers can help deal with experimental design dilemmas in a wide variety of ways. Several of these are outlined below. More details of these and other design options in conjunction with their data analytic requirements can be found in Cook and Campbell's (1979) volume on *Quasi-Experimentation.* A less technical work, but one providing examples drawn from prevention research, is the monograph by Price and Smith (1985).

First Steps

Choosing how to test a theory-based prevention model is a very necessary first step. Unlike laboratory scientists, preventive intervention researchers are usually less at liberty to expect that they will be studying a behavioral outcome that is primarily under the influence of their experimental conditions. As discussed elsewhere, the behavioral etiology of psychopathology and other health problems is complex and often involves complex person–environment transactions shaped by developmental processes over time. There are certainly options among theories on which to build a preventive intervention research study. Those theories that are built on a relatively simple etiologic process are particularly attractive as one can justify ignoring measurement of many other factors that would require measurement in more integrative theories. Such is the case with Gerry Patterson's social learning theory approach to the study of etiology and prevention of conduct disorders. Social learning contingencies applied by parents are the primary variables in his model; individual differences among the children at risk or their parents are accorded much less importance. At the more complex end of the theoretical continuum, for example, is the Jessors' (Jessor & Jessor, 1984) model of adolescent behavioral health where it is also relevant to the prevention of conduct disorders and associated problems of substance abuse, risk taking, and teen pregnancy. It is very attractive to prevention-minded researchers well informed in developmental and clinical literature, since the Jessors point out the complex interplay of many biological, experiential, and environmental factors. Such integrative theories are attractive because they seem to capture the complexities of developmental psychopathology.

The dilemma in selecting a theoretical base for a prevention study then involves choosing between the allure of a well-articulated integrative theory and the power of a more simple, testable one. It is important to recall that the primary purpose of a theory is to be testable so that it is falsifiable. As discussed previously, one can choose to design a project to test for only short links in a longer hypothesized causal chain.

Choosing among True vs Quasi-Experiments

Table 2 shows three categories of research designs. The prevention field is long past tolerating non-experimental designs. Therefore, the choice of a true experiment or one of the quasi-experiments will be determined by one's research hypotheses, the availability of subject groups and intervention contexts, and

Table 2. Types of intervention evaluation research.

Design	Attributes
Pre-experimental	pretest-posttest or posttest only; no control group
Quasi-experimental	pretest-posttest measures; non-equivalent controls or E's as controls; group assignment to conditions
True experimental	pretest-posttest; equivalent intervention and control groups; individual random assignment to groups

institutional and ethical constraints, as well as how much threat to external validity and internal validity is scientifically and politically tolerable.

From my experience, it would seem that preventive intervention research can often combine true and quasi-experiments within a single study. Several of these options are discussed below.

True Experiments—The Elusive Ideal

Random assignment of subjects to different intervention and non-intervention conditions is seen as a key tactic for countering threats to external validity. This is as true for prevention research as it is for other types of studies in which experimental interventions are being tested for effectiveness. Random assignment, however, is often difficult to achieve for a number of pragmatic reasons. First, if the study is conducted in a host institution, it may not be feasible to rearrange the existing grouping and schedules (as is the case with pupils in elementary schools). Second, it may prove counterproductive to argue for true randomization on the grounds of disproving a null hypothesis: No administrator wants to hear that what you are really doing is trying to prove that the "new prevention program" is not any better than no program at all. Institutions or communities planning to host a new prevention program want to be convinced that new preventive interventions will work and will be worth their effort. They also expect to be able to identify those most in need of prevention and to be certain to get them into the intervention group.

For these and other reasons, prevention researchers can rarely hope to conduct time series experiments in real-world settings and time frames. Fortunately, there remain a variety of experimental designs that can be creatively adapted to the needs of prevention researchers. As is pointed out in a later section, the interrupted time-series cross-over group design is a good strategy with which to deal with a number of methodological dilemmas. The point I wish to make here, however, is that prevention researchers should also explore the possible combinations of true and quasi-experimental design elements.

Pressures toward Quasi-Experimentation with Non-Random Assignment to Interventions

The last point touches on a dilemma common to all prevention research, namely, how best to match the potency of a prevention intervention to the levels of risk among the subject target group. It is often true (1) that those most in need of prevention programming are those who may be less capable of responding to it, and (2) that the potency of the preventive intervention may not be equal to the preexisting pressure toward health-risking behaviors. For example, runaway children subsisting on the streets of urban slums are at high risk for substance abuse, sexually transmitted diseases, and psychopathology. Certainly, their need for prevention programs is high. However, the contingencies of their day-to-day survival make it improbable that they can respond positively and enduringly to any prevention program while they remain in the highly pathogenic environment.

Certain quasi-experiments, including the cross-over group design, can employ time and delay of intervention as allies in solving ethical issues involving different levels and sequences of assignment to intervention and non-intervention groups. These designs can be used to reassure participants and cooperating institutions that persons initially assigned randomly to non-intervention-condition groups can be candidates for inclusion in another intervention condition in the future in order to see which works best with whom. Researchers can also honestly advocate that prevention research must constantly evaluate the best means through which to match the potency of intervention with the receptivity of high-risk individuals to preventive intervention. We can borrow from education and clinical treatment traditions of "individualizing" or prescribing different levels of a system approach for subgroups evidencing different constellations of risk factors.

Mass-Targeted vs High-Risk Group-Targeted Prevention Strategies

Mass-targeted prevention research often ignores individual differences when designing or evaluating its interventions. However, not all individuals can be expected to respond equally in an educational or behavioral training program. Some limitations of many mass-targeted prevention applications are as follows:

— Intervention dosage is considered independently of risk status and receptivity.

— Outcome variables are considered non-interactive with
  — individual differences in recipients,
  — individual differences in contexts of intervention,
  — future contexts of expected generationalization effects.

— Reliance on main effects single-factor models.

— Belief that most types of disordered behavior result from the absence of positive skills (mental health status is locatable on a bipolar dimension).

Consequently, there is a great deal of common sense in espousing the notion that mass-targeted programs provide good beginnings to identify broad categories of the population in need for more discriminative prevention research.

Multiple-tracking or *self-selecting procedures* can be built into mass-targeted, randomized subject experimental designs. This might be accomplished by building subject groups with this method:

1) Create intervention assignments through random selection.

2) Create subsequent cohorts with a multiple-gating strategy that employs outcome scores derived from individual responses to a lower cost, mass-targeted preventive intervention.

These scores can be used to determine subsequent assignments to more costly alternative intervention conditions as a function of changes in risk status. An example can be imagined in an adolescent pregnancy prevention program. Pre-adolescents are provided with a mass-targeted sex-education curriculum. Subsequently, early adolescents can be given a second level of intervention involving skills training on how to postpone initiation of intercourse and how to be protected when first

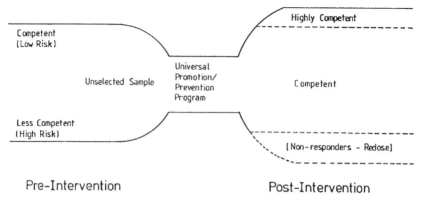

Figure 1. Mass-targeting model of prevention.

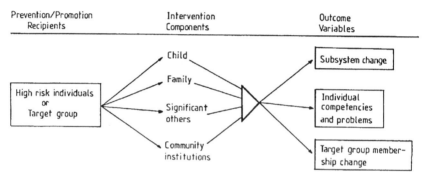

Figure 2. System-oriented model of prevention.

intercourse occurs. A third module of intervention can be tested with already sexually active adolescents. This would provide further contraception training, prevention of STDs, relationship skills, and life planning as it relates to the socioeconomic consequences of childbearing. Such a prevention project would probably require an *interrupted time-series experiment* with both random and prescribed assignment conditions.

Relationship Between Volunteering and Responding to Preventive Intervention Conditions

Given the necessity of conducting prevention research with extremely high-risk patients, can one use self-selection processes as a means for preintervention identification of high-risk subjects who are capable of responding to the potency of the prevention intervention? For example, in designing a preventive intervention research study on street children in Brazil, one can find host institutions providing services to such children who have been motivated to become involved with these service providers. Choosing to study prevention programming effects on the self-selected subjects could be criticized for the inability to generalize research findings to street children in general. However, resorting to random assignment to treatment groups for children not self-selecting to these service providers may, on the other hand, confound the findings with regression on the mean effects and with subjects who are not capable of benefiting from the preventive intervention. A study including both types of subjects in concurrent but still separate subject cohorts would enable the investigator to determine the usefulness of self-selection for determining the type and dosage of preventive intervention. Similarly, one could evaluate the degree to which the responders in each group share characteristics, which might be useful for future recruitments of subjects matched to type and potency of intervention.

Segmenting the Target Population

One should be cautious of certain pitfalls of quasi-experimental designs. One of these is choosing extreme cases for prevention research subjects, which poses a danger of conducting a difficult research project that at best can produce evidence only of a central tendency effect, e.g., where extreme scorers at pretest are likely to have moderate scores at posttest without intervention. Matching for the high initial levels of deviance in the intervention and non-intervention groups does not reduce the risks for regression on the main effects: It will only inform you that your intervention was not necessary.

Unfortunately, social service agencies and political pressures may well require that prevention programs begin with the most visible high-risk groups. Failure to demonstrate positive prevention effects (beyond regression to the mean) with excessively high-risk subjects could jeopardize funding for further research with more moderate-risk subjects who are better suited to the available moderate potency interventions.

Process Evaluation as a Critically Needed Element of Research Design

Process evaluation is an essential part of preventive intervention research. Both outcome and process evaluation can be explicitly designed to identify subgroups of "intervention responders and nonresponders" and subgroups of "intervention compatible and noncompatible" subjects for further planning of new prevention programs. Indeed, the entire prevention process involves recursive cycles as shown by Price and Smith (1985).

Prevention researchers often are not sufficiently trained in nor value the products of process evaluation. Therefore, they can learn a great deal from communication theory and marketing research approaches. Their techniques of process evaluation are particularly relevant to adapting promotion or disease-prevention studies in community contexts.

Guidebooks for Writing Prevention Research Proposals

It would be of help for junior investigators if there were step-by-step guidebooks for writing grants and for choosing among the design options for preventive intervention research. Simple step-by-step questions and suggestions for viable answers can demystify complex issues. I have begun to use such a procedure in teaching preventive research to public health school graduate students. An early draft of one outline of a guide relevant to NIH proposals is appended to this paper.

Strategies to Promote Prevention Research

The goal of preventive intervention research is to demonstrate scientifically effective methods that lead persons at risk for psychopathology and other health problems to develop adequate protective measures. However, because of its complexity, preventive intervention research can be advanced rapidly only on an interdisciplinary basis. New cooperative and synergistic efforts among prevention researchers, training programs, and service providers must be effected.

Several methods are available. They include

1) advocating consciousness raising among policymakers and setting new prevention priorities at funding institutions;

2) creating stable funding for centers engaged in productive research communication, evaluation, and planning;

3) building researcher networks;

4) providing publication outlets;

5) developing training experiences for new investigators.

No single one of these activities can accomplish much without support from the others. While no one type need come first in the sequence, there must be a sequence of activities or their interactive effects will be lost and prevention research will continue to evolve only with painful slowness.

Advocacy for Prevention Research

Just as there is always a need for eloquence in justifying a specific research proposal involving preventive intervention, so can advocacy help in overcoming pervasive prejudices about the prevention field in general. Far too many influential persons in mental health believe that prevention research is premature because there is an inadequate base of epidemiological or etiological studies. These persons tend to view the prevention literature as making a stronger case for its non-definitive soft science methodologies than for its promise as a scientific means to demonstrate how to reduce future incidence of disorders.

On the other hand, prevention researchers would do well to avoid some of the more expansive rhetoric of early prevention advocates. Far too much was promised for many early prevention programs. As Rolf (1985) warned, overpromising what prevention research can deliver in the near future can once again create expectations among policymakers which will be impossible to fulfill. More failures would reinforce pervasive skepticism and may result in future reductions in support for prevention research.

Preventive intervention research is at a disadvantage with respect to its older parent disciplines when it comes to advocacy or lobbying, as it is called in the United States. Prevention researchers, being a professional minority, have weaker voices when it comes to setting either national or local research and fiscal priorities. Its longitudinal and complex implementation designs produce fewer publications and therefore less opportunities for professional advancement. As a member of a minority chorus, prevention researchers are also less socially important within their own parent guilds (e.g., psychiatry or psychology), and they are therefore less likely to reach levels of influence as advisors to research support institutions and governmental regulatory agencies relevant to prevention and health promotion research. There are a number of strategies to help the prevention field to cope with these suppressing realities.

Methods are available to discover how to strike a delicate balance between underselling and overpromising the merits of prevention research. Price and Smith's (1985) recursive diagram of the prevention programming cycle points the way. Communication and marketing theory suggest process research strategies that fit the goals of prevention advocacy as well as they fit the evaluation needs of prevention researchers in the field. An interesting venture for a foundation would be to support a social psychological or marketing approach to assessing how, when, and with what disorders to advocate greater societal support of prevention research. Given the AIDS threat worldwide, this may be the decade and the disease to support major funding for prevention methodological development and intervention trials.

Setting Priorities at Research Support Institutions

Administrators at institutions that fund and promote research and research training often rely on the advice of senior field scientists who are in the more generative and less competitive stage of their careers. Prevention researchers would be well advised to encourage their senior scientists to come forward and gently advocate shifting research funding priorities toward preventive intervention research for specific target populations at risk. This advice should be offered with the understanding that responsible administrators must carefully balance traditional commitments to establish research fields against the need to give special support to a promising but politically less important minority.

Sometimes advocates have won debates over increasing the share for prevention research. And these victories reveal other problems to be solved by the scientists in the field. For example, when advocacy leads to the publishing of new research funding priorities at governmental institutes or private foundations, it serves as a powerful stimulant—though not necessarily a sufficient methods to sustain the desired research activities. This is because new research priorities are often short lived when they do not address the needs of more traditional centers of political influence. This can cause major problems for preventive intervention research as it requires slow start up activities that must be conducted as longitudinal research. Further, the critical mass of investigators usually need to be recruited to the intervention site by someone who does not have alternative sources of salary support beyond the initial grant. For the recruits this means that there are grave risks involved in jumping on a preventive intervention research bandwagon.

For example, it is sad to read in prevention texts (e.g., Roberts & Peterson, 1984; Price & Smith, 1985) of the great promises of a new awakening in the United States of governmental responsibilities to fund prevention research. During the Carter Administration in the United States, a presidential commission on prevention and health promotion produced recommendations that were implemented into a new mental health services law. This new statute contained significantly larger budgetary commitments for prevention and health promotion activities. Unfortunately, with the election of Ronald Reagan a few months later, this law was repealed, and a substitute statute led to cuts in prevention funding.

Sometimes advocacy can produce some programs for prevention researchers which continue to survive even after the political motivation for the initiatives has been replaced by others. For example, the National Institute of Mental Health preventive intervention research center initiative (also begun under the Carter Administration) has produced a number of interdisciplinary research centers throughout the United States. Such a center concept is described below as a very useful technique to promote sustained collaborative research.

Strategies to Get People into the Prevention Research Pipeline

The field needs younger investigators who, through abundant energy and optimism, will see the promise of prevention research more half full than half empty. Youthful investigators are also more likely to have been trained by persons from different backgrounds and disciplines, and are therefore more tolerant of the need to design prevention research with multidisciplinary perspectives and methodologies. However, the life for a new prevention researcher is often less attractive than that available to new professions in more established disciplines. Preventive research is necessarily more risky. Therefore, care must also be taken to assure that there are seasoned investigators to prevent these pioneering young investigators from failing to specify sufficiently short-term dependent variables to enable them to publish and therefore not professionally perish. Several of the more promising strategies are described below.

Strategies for Training New Prevention Researchers

Prevention research, more than most basic, epidemiological, and clinical research, must be an integrative, interdisciplinary field. However, it is very difficult to know how to borrow the very best theories and methods from each of the parent disciplines in designing prevention research. Collective wisdom is often needed to solve the ethical and pragmatic dilemmas of implementing prevention research in field settings. However, it is also a result of inadequate training in intervention research methodology among that small cadre of individuals who are motivated to undertake this difficult research endeavor. The obvious solution is to provide preventive intervention research training in the educational and clinical settings in which the intellectual and technical resources are available to implement prevention research.

Research Training in Preventive Intervention Research

Different disciplinary traditions and types of institutions which train professionals to work in basic, clinical, public health treatment fields have produced an unintegrated body of knowledge as well as have obstructed the creation of interdisciplinary research training programs. Future generations of prevention researchers focusing on discovering ways to alter the etiological chain leading to psychopathology must learn to multiply research methods associated previously with separate disciplines. However, hardly any existing training programs in psychology, psychiatry, or public health reflect the diversity of theories and methods in the growing field of developmental psychopathology and its sister experimental subdiscipline, preventive intervention research.

How can existing programs incorporate the needed multidisciplinary and multi-theoretical perspectives required for prevention research? It seems presently impractical to add courses in developmental psychopathology and preventive intervention methodology to the main training programs in departments of psychology and psychiatry or in some department of a school of public health. Since each type of training institution emphasizes different aspects of psychopathology, what could constitute the best sets of experiences and curricula to train researchers in each setting? How can those inside clinical practice, public health program development, and epidemiology and laboratory studies of human development best inform research training?

Strategies to Promote Collaborative Research

Many traditional research-promoting methods, such as one-time workshops, conferences, and the use of special publication outlets, are too infrequent and episodic to suffice by themselves to accelerate collaborative prevention research. Furthermore, maintaining cooperative research in highly competitive scientific fields is difficult to do very well even for a brief period, let alone for the length of time required for the intensive collaborations needed for prevention studies.

What is needed are innovative means for a rapid increase in rewarding and intellectually productive work among prevention researchers. To move from the creative insights of a handful of researchers to usefully disseminated prevention programs, however, often requires an ongoing series of special meetings and consultations to negotiate new collaborations, to share methods and promising leads, to effect shifts in research project design and staffing arrangements, to create efficient use of network communication systems, and even to help to promote the reallocation of resources of research support institutions into new prevention initiatives.

Fostering Prevention Networks

There is great need for support of an all too rare type of research activity—a working collaborative researcher network—that may be critically important to successful demonstrations of prevention programs in this decade. Traditional research promoting methods based primarily on a competitive model of science (which usually involves secrecy concerning successes and failures prior to publication) are probably not sufficient to accelerate the rate of productive prevention research needed to meet prevention goals. This is certainly true with regard to the increasing threat of HIV infection. An active collaborative network of key prevention researchers and expert consultants is a potent alternative means to move quickly from the creative insights of a handful of researchers to effective and replicable large-scale prevention programs.

The creation of *networks or consortia of researchers* is a difficult but potent method that can quickly promote cooperation and even create a new interdisciplinary field of inquiry (e.g., as was the case with the creation of the field of developmental psychopathology; see Rolf & Read, 1984). Such networking would entail collective problem solving in (a) the creation and testing of prevention modules for persons with different demographic characteristics, (b) cross-project replications of the effectiveness of these modules, (c) consultations on research design, longitudinal assessment, and data analysis, and (d) the indispensable support for continuing with a kind of research known more for its extreme difficulties than its potential to advance the careers of scholar scientists.

A foundation- or government-supported Preventive Intervention Researcher Network could rapidly increase the feasibility and productivity of prevention research by linking key interdisciplinary groups of investigators engaged in prevention research programs with consultants who have complementary expertise, so that they can collectively cope with the complex methodological problems. Such a network would encourage the sharing of promising leads concerning effective prevention methodologies well in advance of their publication in journals or presentations at professional meetings.

A prevention researcher network would also identify and provide the means to link experts needed as consultants by researchers about to begin prevention studies. This is important, because:

1. Prevention research has often been hampered by the fact that those who are willing and better able to recruit subjects in community settings (e.g., schools, neighborhoods, etc.) are not necessarily those best equipped to conduct the rigorously controlled field trials or to undertake the complex longitudinal data analysis procedures.

2. The persons with needed technical expertise in prevention research are rarely locally available to active prevention research projects.

Creating a functioning foundation- or government-sponsored prevention researcher network is not an easy task nor one to be attempted by someone without a long-standing commitment to collaborative research. Its leaders should have relevant experience over the years with regard to fostering communication and collaboration among researchers at different levels of seniority. Certainly the work required to create and maintain the proposed network would be considerable, but there would be people eager to undertake it if there were real promise of sufficient support and commitment by the funding institution. This author's belief in the potential high payoffs from sponsoring cooperative research activities comes from a decade of involvement in the NIMH and Grant Foundation-sponsored "Risk for Schizophrenia Research Consortium," through participation in the creation of the preventive intervention research initiative at NIMH, and especially through my observations of and communications with persons in several of the MacArthur Foundation-sponsored research networks and consortia.

The Prevention Center Strategy

How to bring promising junior investigators together with older, more seasoned prevention veterans has been one of the pressing problems of the preventive intervention research field. What are needed are new and definable strategies to accomplish this goal. Also needed are ways to keep the research team together between grants. Few senior prevention researchers have been able to create a talented prevention research team that has lasted much beyond the limited time frames of research grants or service demonstration programs. (One successful example has been Emory Cowen at Rochester University, who has maintained leadership in applied research and mentoring of junior investigators.) However, it is often the case that having left their mentors, these investigators find that they are all too independent from other similarly motivated individuals to effect a prevention research project. Clearly, what is needed are effective strategies to increase the number of sites where prevention motivation and competence reach critical mass to effect important new studies.

An informative example is the Preventive Intervention Research Centers (PIRC) initiative undertaken by NIMH in 1982. It was designed to promote collaborations among prevention-minded investigators in existing areas of research excellence, even if this excellence was not in prevention research. The intention was to stimulate the creation of interdisciplinary local networks to compete for the more difficult to obtain preventive intervention research grants. The central concept behind the PIRC was to increase the feasibility of good prevention research by linking scientists with complimentary expertise that could then collectively cope with the complex methodological problems inherent in the prevention of mental disorders. Considerable thought and planning went into the writing of the PIRC grant-application guidelines. Included among the criteria for review were the necessity to pay attention to developmental factors, as they were relevant to prospective measurement of the adjustment of high-risk subjects across developmental stages and stressful life transitions. Similarly, persons applying were also to pay attention to how their research timelines and assessment methodology would be adapted to differences among cultural and other types of subgroups within the populations at risk for psychopathology. Following on the model used for funding the already established clinical research centers in the United States, the NIMH guidelines indicated that funding support would be available only for core activities helpful to the network of investigators linked by the PIRC grant. PIRC grant funds were not designed to fund a specific project unless it was a pilot variety. Instead, support was to be dedicated to fostering collaborations and pilot studies that would lead to additional grant proposals for major projects.

With the election of a new president and subsequently the arrival of new heads at the National Institute of Mental Health, the preventive intervention research center effort at increasing generativity came to be perceived as less of a priority than the discovery of more traditional etiological and biomedical and epidemiological research. Today, four PIRC centers survive, and one of our symposium members, Sheppard Kellam, is the head of one of them.

References

Campbell, D., & Stanley, J. (1966). *Experimental and quasi experimental designs in research.* Chicago: Rand-McNally.

Cook, T., & Campbell, D. (1979). *Quasi-experimentation: Design and issues for field settings.* Chicago: Rand-McNally.

Cowen, E. L. (1980). The wooing of primary prevention. *American Journal of Community Psychology, 8,* 258–284.

Garmezy, N., & Rutter, M. (Eds.) (1983). *Stress, coping and development in children.* New York: McGraw-Hill.

Jessor, R., & Jessor, S. L. (1984). Adolescence to young adulthood: A twelve-year prospective study of problem behavior and psychosocial development. In S. A. Mednick, M. Harway, & K. M. Finello (Eds.), *Handbook of longitudinal research in the United States, Vol. 2* (pp. 34–61). New York: Praeger.

Price, R. H., & Smith, S. (1985). *A guide to evaluating prevention programs in mental health.* (DHHS Publications No. (ADM) 85-1365). Washington, DC: Government Printing Office.

Roberts, M. C., & Petersen, L. (Eds.) (1984). *Prevention of problems in childhood.* New York: Wiley.

Rolf, J. (1985). Evolving adaptive theories and methods for prevention research with children. *Journal of Consulting and Clinical Psychology, 53,* 631–646.

Rolf, J., & Read, P. B. (1984). Programs advancing developmental psychopathology. *Child Development, 55,* 8–16.

Zigler, E., & Berman, W. (1983). Discerning the future of early childhood intervention. *American Psychologist, 38,* 894–906.

APPENDIX

Outline for Preparing a Preventive Intervention Research Proposal

I. Begin by creating a summary (abstract) statement of the proposed project. Keep abstract length to one double-sided page. Add more to the abstract as you complete each section below.

A. What is the health problem in need of a preventive program?

B. State what additional research is needed to be able to implement effective prevention programs.

II. What do you intend to do about this need for additional research?

A. Name the overall long-term goal(s) of your project
For example, demonstrate methods to reduce the future incidence of "X" in "Y" kinds of people.

B. State as your *specific aims* the short-term research objectives, including

1. *Intervention innovations* (if you plan on developing the intervention, measures and procedures; see Price & Smith, 1985, Chap. 3): ". . . to develop (age, culturally, etc.) appropriate behavior change prevention curricula . . ."

2. *Process evaluation* (checking on the research steps to find problems with implementation; see Price & Smith, 1985, Chap. 5): ". . . to monitor research activities from recruitment to outcome evaluation to identify procedural barriers and facilitators . ."

3. *Intervention outcome* (behavior changes expected during the research project): ". . . to demonstrate increases in 'z' health-protecting behaviors following intervention . . ."

III. State the *significance* of the targeted problem and previous research background supporting the proposed research.

A. What is the extent of the problem (published incidence and prevalence data if possible)? What are the attendant costs to the individual and to society?

B. What are examples of previous prevention/promotion research applied to this problem? How effective were they?

C. How will the proposed research improve on previous studies and contribute to our scientific knowledge about preventing the targeted problem?

IV. *Research Design.* In this section you will state how you think that this research can be accomplished. It is helpful to begin the section with a brief introductory overview paragraph. You will be able to write this after answering the following key questions:

A. What are your main *hypotheses* to be tested in the proposed research? Specify in terms of your *specific aims* (objectives). Be certain your variables are appropriately listed in Section IV.C.3.a below.
   ". . . . This study proposes to test the effectiveness of 'z' intervention to prevent 'x' in 'y' kinds of subjects. It is hypothesized that ..." (list the hypotheses)

B. What kinds of research design fits this project?
   1. First decide if a true experiment (including random assignment to groups) is feasible.
   2. How much rigorous scientific proof of intervention effects is needed? (Usually, the greater the body of previous prevention research in the targeted problem area, the more rigorous the requirements for additional research.)
   3. What might be the advantages of a "quasi-experimental design"?
      a. Would it increase feasibility?
      b. How can the threats to *external validity* (generalization of findings) and to *internal validity* (potential for errors in sampling, administering, and measuring intervention) be made acceptable? (See Price & Smith, 1985, Chap. 6, and Cook & Campbell, 1979)

C. Next, specify the details of the research methodology. (The questions below concern who gets what intervention, where, how it is given, for how long, how intervention effects [outcomes] are measured, and how the research process is monitored.)
   1. *Subjects* (who gets what intervention)
      a. What type(s) of subjects will be in the study? State

desired demographic characteristics of the re-
searched subjects in need of prevention.

b. How many different types of subject groups will there
be?

1. *Intervention group(s).* Besides the minimum one
experimental intervention group, will there be another kind of intervention group that will receive
a different type or intensity of intervention?

2. *Control group(s).* Will there be one or more control
or (nonequivalent) contrast groups? Be clear about
the purpose of each group and the type of answers
each can provide. How feasible is a study with
multiple groups?

c. How many subjects will be in each group?

1. How many do you think can be managed in the
intervention and contrast conditions at one time?

2. How many subjects will you need to ensure sufficient statistical power to prove or disprove your
hypotheses? (More subjects are needed when the
intervention effects are not expected to be large,
there is not trivial variability of scores within a
group, subject attrition is expected, and a higher
confidence criterion [$p<.01$] is chosen.)

3. Will you need to run a series of several subject
cohorts (waves) to obtain sufficient sample sizes
for your groups?

d. *Draw a subject grid* (chart) with the rows listing the
subject groups and the first column containing the
chosen sample sizes (N's). Use additional columns if
more than one cohort or wave is planned. (Replication experiments at the same or other sites could also
be shown in additional columns.) Make a footnote
explaining if you have allowed for attrition.

e. *Assignment of groups.* How will the subjects be assigned to groups?

1. It's generally best if it can be done randomly. If not
done randomly, explain why not (e.g., ethics, not
permitted by host institution, or other circumstances). Is there any reason to study a self-selected subgroup (as with those who are at very high
risk and probably resistant to intervention target
groups)?

2. Will the groups be intentionally stratified or configured in any way (e.g., to have certain proportions of gender, ages, prior experience, etc.)? Justify your choices.

3. Will matching of subjects between groups be attempted? State your reason and how it will or won't affect outcome measures and generalization.

f. *Subject recruitment.*

1. What kind of recruitment will be necessary to obtain your subject pool (posters, media ads, referrals from an agency, presentations to existing classes in a school)?

2. You may need to detect and correct sampling biases. How will you monitor group composition over time? Will you make replacements or will you start with additional sampling to allow for drop-outs?

2. *Intervention (and non-intervention) conditions and specifications.*

a. Summarize the *basic purpose* and *content* of each intervention.

1. State how each is based on a theory or common sense or both.

2. Will intervention have distinct components (modules)? Here one can include a table outlining the content of the intervention(s) and relate them to the health behaviors to be enhanced or reduced. (A formal grant application would benefit from an appendix providing more detail.)

3. Where (at what site or sites) will intervention be conducted? Will this bias results?

4. Who will give the intervention? Create a staffing list table indicating who will do each job.

5. Will there be standardized procedures? (If not, add comments to "Weaknesses" section below.)

6. What staff training will be necessary prior to and during the intervention phase to ensure adequate and uniform implementation?

b. How long will the intervention(s) last?

1. Will there be a piloting and innovation phase?

2. Does the length of intervention fit reality? Is it enough to have any effects? Do they match the

hypotheses and aims?

3. Sketch a timeline showing the relative lengths of baseline pretests, intervention(s), and posttests. (If required, show or describe how subsequent cohorts or waves of intervention trials fit in the timeline.)

3. *Outcome evaluations*

a. In a table, list the dependent variables and state how each will be measured.

b. It is desirable to have each type of group receive the same measures and assessment schedule. Will this be the case in the proposed study?

1. Pencil in the assessment schedule on the timeline.

2. Have you created any unintended measurement-related threats to internal validity in your assessment plan? Add comments to your "Strengths and Weaknesses Section" below.

c. You'll need to avoid experimenter biases.

1. Be certain to state that dependent variables will not be assessed by those giving the interventions.

2. If behavior ratings are made, to what extent are the ratings made by persons blind to group membership?

d. It's desirable to have several *sources* of information (e.g., from the target subject and an informant) and more than one *type of assessment* (e.g., self-reports, observed performance, etc.). Does the proposed study have a good balance of sources and types of measures?

4. *Process evaluation*

a. What threats to internal validity are evident? What are your methods and how adequate are they for

1. subject recruitment and maintenance?

2. assessment schedules?

3. measurements of dependent variables?

4. implementation of standard intervention and assessment procedures?

b. What is your appraisal of the study's external validity?

1. Can you achieve a true random sampling of the target population?

2. How should one qualify the generalization of findings from the proposed study?

D. *Strengths and weaknesses of the study's design*

1. Start with a general evaluation paragraph.

   a. How adequately does the proposed study address the needed research with important testable hypotheses?

   b. Is your approach adequately based on theory and previous findings?

2. What threats to internal validity are evident?

   a. How adequate are you methods of

     1. subject recruitment and maintenance?

     2. assessment timelines?

     3. measurements of dependent variables?

     4. implementation of standardized intervention and assessment procedures?

3. What is your appraisal of the study's external validity?

   a. To what extent will you be able to generalize to other samples and target populations?

   b. State how you will qualify interpretations of findings according to these limits.

E. *Data management and analyses*

1. *Data management*

   a. Describe how the data management will insure timely, careful, and secure acquisition, coding, readiness for data analyses.

   b. How will confidentiality be assured (e.g., only subject numbers, no identifying information stored with data)?

   c. Indicate who will be responsible for data management (check staffing/budget table).

2. *Data analyses*

   a. State that you will conduct descriptive statistics of the obtained and not obtained (also lost) subjects.

   b. Describe any process evaluation data analyses (e.g., χ^2 of those who completed vs did not like [completed or dropped out of] the program).

   c. Outcome evaluations involve testing for level, immediacy, and duration of intervention effects. State the outcome measures involved and name appropriate statistical analyses (ANCOVA—to partial out an important covariate, like age, IQ; repeated measures ANOVAs, the use of change scores in certain analyses, etc.).

F. *Human subjects*

1. Are there ethical concerns involving the proposed research? Will it involve sensitive topics or potentially harmful procedures?

2. What are the potential benefits to the participants, to society, and to the research staff?

   a. What are the potential risks to participants (subjects and staff)?

   b. What procedures will be effected to minimize them?

      1. Informed consent, right to end participation, protection of confidentiality, referral to alternate service providers when trouble arises, etc.?

   c. To what extent are minors or adults with handicapping/debilitating conditions involved that may limit ability to give informed consent?

   d. What are the legal risks of subject participation (e.g., detection of child abuse, felonies, others)?

G. *References*

List works cited in the body of the proposal. (Note: NIH has placed a 4-page limit on references.)

Prevention Research: The Need for a Realistic Approach

Christian Klicpera

Dr. Rolf addressed three main topics in his paper: the general direction of prevention and prevention research, research design problems, and policies for furthering prevention research. I would like to comment briefly on all three topics, but above all on the first one.

It is still believed that prevention efforts should be especially directed toward primary prevention. I think that Dr. Rolf clarified the limitations of the original conception of primary prevention very well. He correctly pointed out that there is a continuum between primary and secondary prevention that can be understood by placing different intervention efforts on the dimensions of specificity of target groups and specificity of intervention efforts. Especially the notion of three levels of specificity of target groups—general population, normative and non-normative transition stages, risk groups—appealed to me as a very sensible one.

Many transitions carry with them an increased risk and lead to adaptation problems for children and their families. This is even true for many normative transitions, e.g., birth of a new child, entrance to kindergarten, entrance to school and finding a place for vocational training, leaving home. At each of these transitions we find a relatively high percentage of children and families who are not well prepared for this transition. In Vienna, for example, about 10% of the children cannot adapt very well to the transition to primary school and—given a considerable inflexibility of the school system—are removed from their first-grade classes in the first few months. They then attend a preschool program for one year before they can again enter the first grade. The transition from primary to secondary school again is for many children difficult, leading to an increase in behavior and achievement problems. I think that the scheme Dr. Rolf presented sharpens our awareness that intervention at these transition points would be quite fruitful.

A second concept that seems to me as very important is the notion that every intervention is directed onto a system. Thus, we have to consider not only whether an intervention effort is *effective* in itself but also how it *fits into a given system* (e.g., school system). Prevention efforts will not only be more cost-effective when they utilize structures that already exist in the community, but the chance is also much higher that there will be continuity in their implementation after a demonstration project has ended. The question whether to work with existing services and broaden their competencies or to build up new ones is certainly a complicated one that cannot be answered in a general way. School systems, for example, differ in their willingness to let people other than teachers come in and operate a special service. Today, we see in most countries a great willingness to build up special services within schools. But experience has shown that this creates many problems, since all too often the cooperation between these different services and between the services and the teachers doesn't function too well.

Prevention efforts could and probably should also try to rearrange the relative weight given to various goals within given institutions. I think that this has special importance for the school system. In the German-speaking countries at least, there is a widely shared feeling especially among teachers that far too little importance is attached to the social and emotional education of children, in other words, that there is an imbalance between the cognitive and the socio-emotional curriculum (Innerhofer & Klicpera, 1988).

There are many preventive efforts already under way (in the school system, in the youth services, in general social work), programs whose accomplishments and whose functioning have been seldom studied, but which are nevertheless well established. It would be of high priority, in my opinion, to learn more about their way of functioning. The general impression is that many of these prevention efforts are not very effective, but we must know much more than we do now about the factors that impede the initiation of change processes through helping agents.

It is important to study the effectiveness of prevention efforts, though prevention research should not be limited to evaluation research. Research on prevention also means research on health- and adjustment-related change processes in the community. It encompasses basic research on helpful and protective relationships in the social networks and how natural networks are influenced by social policy decisions. It includes basic research on the internalization of values, on the technology of social education, on the work of social institutions, and on the implementation of social policies (Brandstätter, 1982).

Prevention research would be more acceptable to many institutions if evaluation were combined with a detailed study of the intervention process with the aim of improving the existing services.

As far as evaluation research is concerned, I think that it would be important to combine qualitative and quantitative research methods (Cronbach, 1975). All too often research reports fail to tell us anything about how the intervention is *perceived* by the target groups. How do they describe their experience with the prevention program, what meaning do they attach to these experiences? Verbatim statements would sometimes be more useful than standardized questionnaires in understanding the impact of the prevention program (Campbell, 1979).

The goals for an intervention should be formulated in a very specific way. The same is true for the rationale behind any intervention effort. The theory on which an intervention is based should be explicit and specific, and it should be based on empirically derived knowledge about the development of deviant/maladjusted behavior. If such a theory includes too many unknown or too few explored variables, we are probably not ready for an effective intervention program and for research on it.

A few words on the second topic addressed by Dr. Rolf—research design problems. There are some other threats to the validity of an intervention which he didn't mention or at least didn't stress enough, in my opinion, and which seem to be very important:

— Is the treatment actually carried out as it was supposed to be carried out?

— How does the intervention affect other parts of the system in which it is implemented? When an intervention takes place, for example, in a school, what is going on in the class while some children from the same class participate in a special training or therapy program?

— Is the treatment in the context of an institution not transformed into something which was not intended?

Prevention research probably will not make much progress by single, isolated studies; there should be plans for a research program in which studies build upon each other. That any prevention program is effective or is not effective doesn't tell us too much. We must have much more knowledge about the change processes that are initiated by the program, the conditions under which the operation of such a program is effective, and so on.

A last question I would like to ask, although this has already been mentioned by Dr. Wolkind during the discussion: What should be the role of child psychiatry as a *profession* in the process of prevention? I see a danger in stretching the competencies too far. Maybe the main role of child psychiatry should be within the health field: alerting other health professions/health specialists; getting those who work within the health field to cooperate.

The role child psychiatrists could and should play depends certainly on the quality of existing lines of cooperation with other professional fields (education, social workers and so on). It also depends on whether the child psychiatrist can abstain from trying to dominate other professions by relying on the predominant role of the medical model in our society. I think there is a danger as well as a chance, because the high awareness of health-related issues in our society can also be a chance, for example, for setting up centers for research on prevention. It depends very much on finding the right balance.

References

Brandstätter, J. (1982). Methodologische Grundfragen psychologischer Prävention. In J. Brandstätter & A. von Eye (Eds.), *Psychologische Prävention: Grundlagen, Programme, Methoden.* Bern: Hans Huber.

Campbell, D. T. (1979). Degrees of freedom and the case study. In D. T. Cook & C. S. Reichardt (Eds.), *Qualitative and quantitative methods in evaluation research.* Beverly Hills, CA: Sage.

Cronbach, L. (1975). Beyond the two disciplines of scientific psychology. *American Psychologist, 30,* 116–127.

Innerhofer, P., & Klicpera, C. (1988, in press). *Integration und Schulreform. Eine Untersuchung zur Integration Behinderter an den Pflichtschulen Südtirols.* Heidelberg: Schindele.

Barriers to Implementation of Research Findings

Philip Graham

It is unusual to consider it necessary to discuss the reasons why research findings so often fail to be applied to the benefit of children and their families. Yet this subject is quite possibly the most important to be discussed in the symposium. For there may be little point in advancing the frontiers of knowledge if such knowledge is not being properly applied. Let us consider the degree to which this is true, and then go on to consider why such knowledge is not implemented. The reasons vary:

1. *Severe mental retardation.* About one-third of all babies with this condition suffer from Down Syndrome (Tizard, 1964). We can now detect this condition by amniocentesis, and the pregnancy can be terminated when a positive result is obtained. There is no scientific reason why such a policy should not be adopted in all pregnancies, but it is, of course, more cost-effective in older women. The fragile-X-syndrome, the recessive sex-linked disorder responsible for about 10% of all severe mental retardation in boys (Bundey et al., 1985), could be prevented in the same way or, alternatively, amniocentesis could be restricted to subsequent pregnancies in women who had already given birth to an affected child. Thus, it would be possible, with these two measures alone, to reduce the rate of severe mental retardation by about 35–40%.

2. *Mild mental retardation* (MMR). Though genetically determined conditions such as the fragile-X-syndrome are responsible for a higher proportion of the condition than was once thought to be the case (Thake et al., 1987), most mild mental retardation is probably due to inadequate and/or insensitive stimulation. Children at risk for mild mental retardation, i.e., those born to young, isolated women living in deprived circumstances, could probably nearly all be reared to achieve a level of average ability by programs of continuous enrichment or by adoption (Clarke & Clarke, 1984; Seglow et al., 1972). It is not possible to estimate the degree to which mild mental retardation could be prevented by such measures, but certainly the effect would be considerable. If a significant reduction in the level of MMR led to a restandardization of intel-

ligence tests, there would, of course, still be a roughly similar number of children scoring two standard deviations or more below the mean, but the positive effect on the functional level of retarded children would remain a real one. Alternatively, the implementation of social and economic programs to reduce poverty and improve housing would probably have a powerful indirect effect on rates of mild mental retardation.

3. Conduct disorders and emotional disorders specific to childhood. We know that marital disharmony is related to these conditions, and there is a strong likelihood that the effect is causal (Quinton & Rutter, 1985). Thus, if parents were able to settle their differences amicably and to rear their children in a consistent, sensitive manner, there is evidence that the rate of these disorders would reduce, though it is uncertain to what degree. We also know (Rutter et al., 1979) that if the atmosphere in schools were pervaded by an academic ethos, if teachers turned up regularly for lessons, set and marked homework regularly, distributed responsibility among a number of their pupils rather than concentrating it on very small numbers, and if they exercised reward for good behavior rather than punishment for bad, rates of conduct and emotional disturbances in school would probably remit. Again, the size of the effect is uncertain. Successful interventions of both a group and individual nature have also been demonstrated (Kolvin et al., 1981) to have the effect of reducing the rates of psychiatric disorder in children of school age.

4. *Enuresis.* If the work of Brazelton (1962) is to be taken at face value, child-centered counseling of parents concerning the toilet training of their children would drastically reduce the rate of nocturnal enuresis.

Now, even with existing knowledge, there are some child psychiatric and developmental disorders we have little idea how to prevent. Childhood autism and anorexia nervosa are examples of these. The hyperkinetic syndrome is probably another, although there are those who would see the removal of additives and preservatives from purchasable food (Feingold, 1975) and the elimination of lead from petrol (Needleman et al., 1979) as being steps in this direction. The evidence that these measures would make a real difference is, in fact, equivocal (Smith et al., 1983; Cant, 1986). Nevertheless, if scientific knowledge were the sole consideration, it is clear that, given the state of existing knowledge, many disorders are indeed preventable. Why then are they not prevented?

Reasons for Failure of Implementation of Research Findings

Culturally Determined Patterns of Behavior

Parental Rights

The degree to which children are regarded as parental posses-
sions that parents may treat as they wish varies from country
to country and from time to time. In some societies, there are
virtually no restrictions on the degree to which parents may
show cruelty, violence, and neglect to their children; in others,
parents are seen not to own their children, but merely to have
children's welfare in their trust (Nicholson, 1986). If they are
seen to abuse or betray this trust, then their children can be
taken away. As a matter of practice, there are no societies in
which it is made easy to remove children from parental care,
except in extreme cases.

The Right of the Foetus to Life

In some societies, there are strongly held views that, from the
moment children are conceived, they are individuals with a
right to survival, even if the evidence is that they will be severely
handicapped at or after birth; in others, arbitrary points at
different stages of the pregnancy or at birth are considered to
mark the point at which a child has an unequivocal right to
survive.

The Sanctity of Biological Parenthood

Whereas in most Western countries, adoption or long-term
foster care are regarded as feasible options when parental care
breaks down irretrievably, in Muslim societies this practice is
forbidden.

Lack of Knowledge

Social and Economic

There is no agreement on ways in which reduction of poverty and improvement in living standards might be achieved. For example, the British government currently takes the view that economic growth and the relief of poverty are most likely to occur as a result of tax reform, reducing the standard rate of tax and thus releasing resources for private investment. Their political opponents, in contrast, believe that any additional resources should be specifically directed toward increasing benefits to the poor, providing housing subsidies, etc. The decisions that are taken in this respect are vital to the welfare of children, yet it is clear that—bearing in mind that both government and opposition parties believe they are behaving in the best interests of children—there are no clear indications as to which policy would be most likely to achieve this end.

Organizational Rigidity

It may be true that, if all secondary schools were as good as the rest, there would be lower rates of behavior and emotional disorders in children attending these. However, although the research unit at the Institute of Psychiatry, London, continues to pursue this area, it has not yet been possible to demonstrate feasible solutions to the problems of organizational change. It is generally thought that the leadership characteristics of head teachers hold the key to the problem, yet the best methods of selecting head teachers and the strategies they should adopt to change the running of their schools in the right direction are unknown. The attempts the present British government are making both to increase parental involvement in choice of school and in obtaining greater control over the curriculum may have an indirect effect on rates of behavior and emotional disorder through their influence on these factors, though the direction of this influence is uncertain.

Amounts of Explained Variance

Although there are many examples of significant association between rates of emotional and behavior disorder and adverse factors in the background, the amount of variance explained by these factors is often disappointingly small. Thus, the children of parents with disharmonious marriages have about twice the rates of those whose parents have harmonious marriages (Richman et al., 1982), but the great majority of children whose parents have disharmonious marriages are not disturbed. The same holds true for other variables such as maternal depression, poor housing, etc., that have been related to rates of child psychiatric disorders. Herculean efforts to improve family relationships might therefore only have marginal effects on total population rates of disorder.

Inappropriate Professional Training

The training of many professionals dealing with child health problems appears inappropriate to this task and fails to equip them for the real world in which knowledge changes and new techniques are found to be more appropriate than traditionally taught methods. Thus, research findings on intervention are unlikely to be implemented if they suggest behavioral management is effective when a generation of professionals, especially in the social work field, have been trained to believe that behavioral management techniques are usually inappropriately applied and merely lead to symptom substitution. Professionals trained to believe, on the basis of what is probably a misinterpretation of the writings of Bowlby (1951), that day-care centers and nursery schools are harmful to young children because they create artificial separations, find it difficult to reverse their views when new evidence emerges.

Poor Dissemination of Knowledge

McCall and Gregory (1982) have pointed to the lack of enthusiasm many research workers show for communicating via the mass media. Yet if changes in policy and practice do not come about on the basis of research findings alone, but also because of changes in the climate of public opinion, it is surely important for those research workers interested in the implementation of their findings to take what opportunities they can to influence public opinion.

Lack of Commitment to the Needs of Children

It is difficult to bring firm evidence to bear on the issue of political and social commitment, but there are strong arguments for suggesting that, when considering why action for children on the basis of established knowledge is not taken, one reason may lie in the low priority given to the need for such action. When, as has happened in the U.K., child benefit is selectively removed from the list of index-linked benefits despite knowledge of the links between poverty and impaired child development, government must be seen as placing the need for a budget surplus over the needs of children. When teachers undertake industrial action for higher pay and reduce school activities involving parent-teacher communication for months at a time, they can readily be seen as putting their own needs ahead of those of children. When parents of young children cannot resolve their differences without constant strife or separation, they are again surely putting their own needs before those of their children. Although politicians, teachers, and parents would doubtless deny any lack of commitment to the needs of children and would argue how their actions are indeed in favor of the needs of children rather than against them, an impartial observer might yet remain sceptical.

Lessons from Research Findings That Have Been Implemented

What lessons are to be learnt from research finding that *have* been implemented? It might be thought that it would be difficult to identify any situations in which this has occurred, but this would in fact be too negative a view. Examples of research findings implemented on a large scale include:

1. The closing down or very considerable reduction of hospital beds for the mentally handicapped on the basis of findings that children fare better when living at home or in small group hostels.

2. The removal of lead from petrol on the basis of findings of lowered IQ in children with high levels of tooth lead.

3. The use of low phenylalanine diets in children with phenylke- tonuria on the evidence of brain damage occurring as a result of exposure to hyperphenylalanaemia.

4. Reduction in the use of food additives and preservatives on the basis of the findings that these increase hyperactivity.

5. Reduction of bullying in Norwegian schools (Olweus, 1987).

There are also a number of measures that have been taken in which research findings have been supportive to change, but in relation to which other factors have been of probably greater importance in ensuring policy change. These include:

1. Reduced use of high-rise accommodation to house families with young children.

2. Integration of handicapped children into mainstream educa- tion.

3. Greater awareness of the needs of isolated mothers, their proneness to depression, and the inappropriateness of anxi- olytic and antidepressive medication with a drop in the use of psychotropic medication and an increase in part-time em- ployment.

This is not an exhaustive list, and the policies included and not included in it are open to argument, but perhaps *some lessons can be learnt by examining it:*

1. The likelihood that a measure will be implemented does not depend on the quality of the scientific research underpinning it. The work on lead in petrol and on the effects of food additives and preservatives, for example, is controversial and open to numerous methodological objections. In contrast, methodologically satisfactory studies examining effects of schools and family life have been ignored. Only very occa- sionally, as with the work of Olweus (1987), does widespread intervention occur on the basis of sound methodological re- search.

2. The findings of scientific research are more likely to be implemented if their conclusions are consistent with an al- ready existing philosophy tending in the same direction, i.e., if scientists produce findings the public is ready to listen to, they are more likely to be heard.
   A fortiori, it may be noted that research findings will be even more rapidly acted on if there is a strong, popular movement

in their favor. The educational integration of handicapped children and the campaign for lead-free petrol are examples.

3. Findings that indicate a simple cause-effect relationship, e.g., high blood phenylalanine levels causing mental retardation, are more likely to be implemented. Those that reflect complex multi-causal relationships are more likely to be ignored. Thus, findings that reflect the complexity of the way in which disturbed family relationships affect children and findings that threaten already well-established organizations like ordinary schools are less likely to be implemented.

These conclusions may seem rather depressing to research workers who see their work as distinctly less valuable unless it impinges on social policy. In my view, such disappointment is only allowable to those research workers naive enough to believe that their work carries such high status as to justify immediate translation into action. To others, these conclusions may indeed produce reflection on ways in which research workers might tackle their tasks and disseminate their results, but carries no message for discouragement. We do need, however, to consider more systematically how the various barriers to implementation of research findings can be tackled.

Overcoming Barriers to Implementation of Research Findings

Socio-Cultural Practices, Beliefs, and Attitudes

Interestingly, attitudes and beliefs in relation to children have been rather little studied, though the volume of relevant work carried out by sociologists (Jenks, 1985) and social historians of the family has increased very considerably over the past 15 years. There has, however, been very little indication of the way in which such attitudes change or may systematically be changed. We know that change does occur, but the reasons for change remain obscure. Some research workers (e.g., Rees, 1987) believe that empirical social research should include a political dimension with investigation, for example, of the way the role of gate-keepers to social change may be influenced with regard to the policies under investigation. The investigations of beliefs in the population concerning means of disciplining children in relation to child abuse has been discussed elsewhere (Graham et al., 1985).

Organizational Rigidity

Adequate discussion of means of achieving organizational change in schools and other institutions caring for children, such as day care and residential centers, presents a considerable task not to be attempted here; but there is a literature on the subject that borrows many concepts from business management. The importance of leadership, clearly defined objectives with strategies to meet these objectives is frequently emphasized. Investigations inspired by the studies of Rutter and his colleagues demonstrating the importance of schools and the way schools change have not so far produced generalizable results, although it is difficult to estimate the impact of such widely publicized research, and the effects may be greater than the published literature suggests. Jointly funded Health and Education Department projects would seem to be an appropriate way of tackling this type of subject, because while health professionals may be involved in helping to set goals, educationalists will have to find the strategies and resources to effect change; and unless both groups of professionals are motivated for this task, its chances of success will be smaller. Further, intervention that is multilevel, aimed at head teachers, classroom teachers, children, and parents, may have a greater chance of successful implementation than more narrowly focused forms of intervention (Olweus, 1987). Further, interventions are likely to be more widely practiced if those who have developed them undertake dissemination themselves. For example, workshops for primary health care workers, such as health visitors and child health clinic doctors, in the treatment of sleep disorders, organized by Richman and Douglas (1982), have been significantly successful in the implementation of interventions developed for this purpose.

Training Barriers

The need for professionals in the health, social work, and educational fields who can be both thoughtfully critical and positively responsive to research findings has already been mentioned. Regrettably, in all these fields, research findings are often unknown, ignored, or dismissed if they come to notice, in favor of traditionally held views. Sheldon (1987) has described a series of seminars held jointly between research workers and practicing social workers aiming to overcome these problems. In each seminar there was a focus on fields of study in which there had been recent advances that might not yet be known to the service staff—effectiveness and client opinion being prime candidates for inclusion. Each session began with a review of conventional understanding and proceeded to delineate new developments. Staff were not spared discussions of methodological questions. The implications of new research for practice were clearly spelled out. A debate was encouraged on obstacles to the implementation of new findings. Written summaries of the main arguments for each session were available for participants to take away and study. Finally, academic staff agreed to act as consultants on any new projects arising from the series. Sheldon (1987) reports many positive side effects from joint seminars of this type both for the research workers and for the service staff. He also reports the possibility of using objective outcome measures to assess their effectiveness. Indicators such as attendance rates at the seminars, the degree of active participation by members, and rate of borrowing from the departmental library are examples. Such seminars might be even more effective if they were multidisciplinary in nature, thus providing the opportunities for professionals from different disciplines to learn from each other, appreciate the special problems each discipline faces, and enhancing mutual respect.

Dissemination of Information to the General Population

Much research is commissioned by grant-giving bodies whose funds are raised from general taxation. There is therefore a very real sense in which the public has a right to be informed of the results of research: it is paying for it. Further, as has already been suggested, research findings are more likely to be implemented if the policies they suggest are supported by public opinion. Such opinion is more likely to be well informed if serious attempts are made to disseminate findings. Many research professionals are suspicious of the media as a vehicle for communication. They believe, not without some justification, that the media tend to get things wrong, tend to focus on lively personalities rather than on relevant issues, are more concerned about the newsworthiness of findings than their methodological validity, and are little troubled by adverse effects their reporting might produce on the population. McCall and Gregory (1982) have discussed the degree to which these views are unfounded, and suggested ways in which professionals might communicate through the media more effectively. The number of responsible journalists is certainly much greater than many professionals are prepared to accept.

Positive Messages

One major problem relating to implementing research findings concerns the degree to which findings carry few implications beyond the communication of despair. When one has read a series of articles about the effects of maternal depression, disharmonious family relationships, adverse temperamental characteristics, chromosome abnormalities, and cerebral dysfunction, one may be left with a strong sense of impotence and little impetus to action. In contrast, studies reporting protective mechanisms, coping strategies, and the implementation of effective interventions leave one more hopeful and perhaps more prepared for positive activity. Trends toward the investigation of such positive aspects of child mental health (Rutter, 1981) are most welcome and deserve continuing priority.

Directions of Research

If, as seems to be the case, particularly in the first 5 years of a child's life, family functioning is both central to healthy personality development and difficult to alter, then perhaps research should be focused as a priority on the interface between the family and the outside world. Such studies might make it easier for the families to function effectively, even if no direct attempt were make to influence the way they function. Such studies might include examination of ways of improving support for parents, especially mothers, through economic benefits, fiscal measures, personal social support, improving neighborhood cohesiveness, enhancing parent-teacher or parent-nursery group communication, and doubtless in many other ways. Studies that examine positive strategies for improvement should be preferred to those specifically highlighting deficits or parental inadequacies.

Conclusions

An examination of the barriers to implementation of research findings suggests that, although many research findings have not been implemented, some (not necessarily the most impressive ones) have met a better fate. Lessons can be learnt from circumstances in which findings have led to significant action. These include the need to take into account and perhaps investigate cultural beliefs and attitudes. The built-in institutional rigidity of organizations such as schools must be acknowledged. Improved methods of multi-disciplinary training and communication through the media are required. Positive messages are easier to implement than negative ones. Finally, it is suggested that, if research implementation is to be a major consideration in determining research priorities, then studies examining the interface between the family and the outside world may have the greatest promise.

References

Bowlby, J. (1951). *Maternal care and mental health.* Geneva: WHO.

Brazelton, T. B. (1962). A child-oriented approach to toilet training. *Pediatrics, 29,* 121–128.

Bundey, S., Webb, T., Thake, A. J., & Todd, J. (1985). A community study of severe mental retardation in the West Midlands, and the importance of the fragile X syndrome in its aetiology. *Journal of Medical Genetics, 22,* 258–266.

Cant, A. (1986). Diagnosis and management of food allergy. *Archives of Diseases in Childhood, 61,* 730–731.

Clarke, A. M., & Clarke, A. D. B. (1984). Social influences in the aetiology and prevention of mental retardation. In J. Dobbing (Ed.), *Scientific studies in mental retardation.* London: Macmillan.

Feingold, F. B. (1975). Hyperkinesis and learning difficulties linked to artificial food and colors. *American Journal of Nursing, 75,* 797–803.

Graham, P., Wolkind, S., & Dingwall, R. (1985). Research issues in child abuse. *Social Science and Medicine, 21,* 1217–1228.

Jenks, C. (1982). *The sociology of childhood.* London: Batsford.

Kolvin, I., Garside, R. F., Nicol, A. R., Macmillan, A., Wolstenholme, F., & Leitch, I. M. (1981). *Help Starts Here: The maladjusted child in the ordinary school.* London: Tavistock.

McCall, R. B., & Gregory, T. G. (1982). Communicating developmental research to the general public. In J. de Wit & A. L. Benton (Eds.), *Perspectives of child study.* Lisse: Swets and Zeitlinger.

Needleman, H., Gunnoe, C., Leviton, A., Reed, R., Peresie, H., Maher, C., & Barrett, P. (1979). Deficits in psychologic and classroom performances of children with elevated dentine lead levels. *New England Journal of Medicine, 300,* 689–695.

Nicholson, R. (1986). *Ethics of research in children.* Oxford: Oxford University Press.

Olweus, D. (1987). *Aggression in the schools: Effects of a nationwide intervention program.* Paper presented at the American Academy of Child Psychiatry Meeting in Washington, USA, October 1987.

Quinton, D., & Rutter, M. (1985). Family pathology and child psychiatric disorder: A four year prospective study. In R. Nicol (Ed.), *Longitudinal studies in child psychology and psychiatry* (pp. 91–134). Chichester: Wiley.

Rees, S. (1987). The culture-bound state of evaluation: Implications for research and practice. *British Journal of Social Work, 17,* 645–660.

Richman, N., & Douglas, J. (1982). *Sleep Management Manual.* Department of Psychological Medicine, Hospital for Sick Children, London.

Richman, N., Stevenson, J., & Graham, P. (1982). *Pre-school to school: A behavioural study.* London: Academic Press.

Rutter, M. (1981). Stress, coping and development. *Journal of Child Psychology and Psychiatry, 22,* 323–356.

Rutter, M., Maughan, B., Mortimore, P., & Ouston, J. (1979). *Fifteen thousand hours.* London: Open Books.

Seglow, J., Kellmer Pringle, M., & Wedge, P. (1972). *Growing up adopted.* Slough: NFER.

Sheldon, B. (1987). Implementing findings from social work effectiveness research. *British Journal of Social Work, 17,* 573–586.

Smith, M., Delves, T., Lansdown, R., Clayton, B., & Graham, P. (1983). The effects of lead exposure on urban children. *Developmental Medicine and Child Neurology, Suppl. 47.* London: Spastics International Medical Publications.

Thake, A., Todd, J., Webb, T., & Bundey, S. (1987). Children with the fragile X syndrome at schools for the mildly mentally retarded. *Developmental Medicine and Child Neurology, 29,* 711–719.

Tizard, J. (1964). *Community services for the mentally handicapped.* London: Oxford University Press.

From Prevention to Promotion

Ingrid Spurkland

Professor Graham has given a very clear and good overview of the given subject. It would be natural to simply agree with his evaluations. I will, however, give some supplementary comments, to highlight what I think are important points. One of them is economy.

Research is expensive. Programs set up for implementation of research findings may be very expensive. Programs directed toward the general public may be prohibitively expensive.

In Norway, as in most other Western countries, our health and welfare budget has increased dramatically during the last decades. We have reached the point where we cannot expect further increases. Our politicians are unyielding on this: Further development in these areas must rely upon a redistribution of existing funds. We cannot expect to have our budget increased at the expense of, for instance, the education or transport budget—not to mention the defence budget.

These are hard realities for us who work with children and adolescents, and even more so when the concern is children's mental health. It cannot be denied that psychiatry has less status—less general appeal—than somatic medicine. We are faced with having to compete with our somatic colleagues for our piece of the "economic pie," and treatment still has priority before prevention. Arguments for increased funds in our field have to be good—they must be based on well-grounded, coherent knowledge. Preferably, we should be able to present a clear cause-and-effect relationship. It is characteristic that we have received most support for the prevention of mental illness in conditions involving chromosome and enzyme defects. In other words, in conditions more related to somatic medicine than to psychiatry.

As the struggle for adequate funding becomes more difficult, new attention-getting methods are being used. We see more and more how the economic resources are being governed by diverse pressure groups through the mass media. The fashion now is AIDS and heart surgery.

How can the politicians deal with contradictory messages, sift out pertinent information and put it into reasonable perspective? Which professionals can they trust to present careful and objective data that form a sound basis for decisions? Do some of these experts have ulterior motives? Or, how can politicians resist the pressures of public opinion and its demands for financing the one or another project, without risking diminished popularity?

Politicians have to relate to economic realities. They must make choices. But often one feels that it is the "middle-aged men's need for heart surgery" that is the guiding principle in this decision making. The total picture—the comprehensive viewpoint—shines through only by virtue of its absence.

In the competition for our share of the budget for financing mental health and welfare programs, child psychiatry will not obtain what we know to be necessary.

Nevertheless, the situation is not as gloomy as it may appear. Professor Graham stressed that it is easier to implement research findings through positive strategies than through negative ones. To generalize: One can see here a distinction between prevention of disease and promotion of health. Prevention of disease is associated with the identification of risk factors and the initiation of programs for risk groups. Promotion of health concerns the entire population.

Promotion of mental health is both challenging and ambitious. It assumes that "good health" can be defined, as well as which qualitative factors are important. Probably, within a given society, it will be easier to come to an agreement here, than deciding how the goal may be achieved.

By transferring attention from prevention of disease to promotion of health, however, our stake in the national budget becomes different. Instead of fighting for the increase of a small sub-sub-chapter of the budget, we may get in a better position for influencing the greater part of it.

Another barrier for implementation of knowledge is this: Not only mental and physical *illness*, but also mental and physical *health*, have been regarded either as an individual responsibility, or as the doctors' and hospitals' responsibility. We are put into this role and we accept it very easily. This raises the ethical problem, who has the right to define what is good and beneficial for other people? This could by itself be the subject of a symposium. Since health is influenced by the physical and social environment, it becomes important not to monopolize the field. On the contrary, we must insist on cooperation and bring forward the fact that good health is a *common* responsibility. It concerns everyone—teachers, architects, and city planners—to the same degree, and perhaps even more, than it concerns health personnel.

Talking about health, we usually use terms suggesting *illness*; morbidity, disability, risk behavior and hospital admittance are some examples. In this way associations related to health tend to be negative, for instance, anti-smoking campaigns that become scare propaganda. It will therefore be important to define parameters implying the positive qualities of the word "health."Identifying children at risk is *not* the greatest problem. We know a good deal about risk factors. As has been mentioned several times during these days, the interesting question is *why* some children manage despite unfortunate circumstances? What characterizes the "good copers" in a risk group? Which coping strategies have these children developed? Which are the resilient factors? Rutter points out that attention must be given to key turning points in the life span, when the opportunities exist for an alteration of a risk trajectory to a path of resilience (Rutter, 1986). This is an interesting and optimistic point of view and needs further investigation.

We now have both extensive and more limited intervention programs that are directed toward supporting child development. From experiences with these, we have learned a great deal. Graham mentioned Kolvin and associates' work with school children (Kolvin et al., 1981). Others have been working with the lower age groups through their "caretakers"; for example, Barker's Child Development Programme in England, and Sommerschild's community based program in one of Oslo's suburbs (Barker, 1986; Sommerschild, 1987).

Sommerschild trained lay people to run parents groups as an integral part of the Child Care and Welfare Clinics. In Norway, these clinics are utilized by 95% of all families with preschool children. Young parents, broken marriages, often combined with poor social networks, are factors that weaken the natural passing over from generation to generation of values and norms pertinent to child-raising. The groups aimed to compensate for lost mutual exchange of experiences, and they had no educational goal. The program, open to everybody in order to avoid stigmatization of particular parents, was based in a local area and maintained stability over years. These facts contributed to the success of the project. The groups increased the parents' self-confidence and self-esteem, and gave a sense of meaningful solidarity. Measures for improving the environmental milieu for children and adolescents are, by their very nature, multifaceted and complex. The research findings, when looked at separately, have a weak persuasive effect. We therefore need a series of projects that support and supplement each other. Similarly, the research must as far as possible be related to the social context where the findings are meant to be realized. Otherwise, implementation of our research results can risk being rejected as "irrelevant for us." Several attempts to bring forth community diagnoses, in order to initiate preventive programs, are now in progress. This brings me back to health as a common responsibility.

The Healthy Cities Project under the direction of the World Health Organization is an important and exciting program that is working towards these goals. In 1986, European cities were invited to join in a cooperative project that could:

— "Put health high on the political agenda of city politics,

— put health promotion policy an integral part of city policy,

— challenge the health bureaucracy of the city to transgress boundaries and work with other sectors of city government,

— involve citizens of all ages, races and of either sex,

— build a new health culture through new types of projects and coalitions,

— develop a public debate on health in the city that lays open problems, inequalities and constraints for action" (Hancock & Duhl, 1987).

The concept of a healthy city is a very ambitious and extensive one. It will carry different meanings to each separate nation, city and culture. The definition of a healthy city may be one that focuses on the *process* rather than on a final condition.

The challenge of the Healthy Cities Project is its radical break with the general understanding of the nations' health being solely a medical question. Herein lies a possibility to overcome the barrier I mentioned previously: our profession's tendency to monopolize both disease and health. Health, both somatic and mental, is primarily a question of lifestyle. It is deeply affected by attitudes, norms, and values. From a historical perspective, we know that medical progress has only a minor effect on the improvement of health. Possibly, social and economic improvements have been much more influential. The parents are the architects of the family and their well-being is of the greatest importance to their children. Therefore, it is probable that a general improvement of the adults' quality of life and standard of living will have a strong positive effect on the children. This should inspire us to a far greater degree to collaborate with professionals within other areas of our society, both in order to provide new knowledge, to study *methods* of prevention, and to *initiate* implementation of the knowledge we already have, while the carrying through of *general* preventive programs is not necessarily our task.

References

Barker, W. (1986). Child Development Programme, a series of publications from Early Child Development Unit. University of Bristol.

Hancock, T., & Duhl, L. (1987). *Healthy cities: Promoting health in the urban context.* Geneva: WHO, Regional Office for Europe.

Kolvin, I., Garside, R. F., Nicol, A. R., Macmillan, A., Wolstenholme, F., & Leitch, I. M. (1981). *Help starts here: The maladapted child in the ordinary school.* London/New York: Tavistocks Publications.

Rutter, M. (1986). Child psychiatry: Looking 30 years ahead. *Journal of Child Psychology and Psychiatry, 27,* 803–840.

Sommerschild, H. (1987). Prevention in child psychiatry. *Acta Psychiatrica Scandinavica, 76* (Suppl. 337), 59–63.

Author Index

Subject Index

DATE DUE